RESTORE the BODY GOD GAVE
YOU and **FEEL GREAT AGAIN!**

# Heal YOUR Cells.
# SAVE
# YOUR
# LIFE!

## DR. GORDON
## CROZIER

**F** FREILING
PUBLISHING

Published by Freiling Publishing,
a division of Freiling Agency, LLC.

70 Main Street, Suite 23-MEC
Warrenton, VA 20186

www.FreilingPublishing.com

**Library of Congress Control Number: 2019910087**

ISBN 9781950948086

Printed in the United States of America

To Michelle, for her love and enduring support

# Acknowledgements

There are so many people who helped make this book possible. First and most importantly, I want to thank my wife Michelle who encouraged me to leave my teaching career at the University and to find my true passions, which resulted in our important work together at Crozier Clinic. She has been an incredible source of strength for me and for our entire staff. I also want to thank Tom Freiling for helping me accomplish my dreams and aspirations as well as helping to publish books that have helped so many people, and also many thanks to my amazing editor Christen M. Jeschke. I thank my friend, the amazing entrepreneur Steve Scott for his encouragement along the way. I'm also grateful to my peers and to those who have paved the way for a better understanding and acceptance of non-traditional medicine including Dr. Daniel Amen, Dr. Jim LaVelle, Dr. Yan Trokel, and Dr. Joseph Cleaver. I could not begin to thank all the individuals who have aided in helping me attain more knowledge at A4M and IFM. My pastor and his wife, Ron and Sandy Johnson, are my spiritual foundation and deserve much thanks. Also many thanks for my friends Stan and Kathryn Turk.

Lastly, but most important, I am so grateful for all the people around the world who trust me with their health. I love my patients! Let us all keep the quest for what is scientific and the true cause of disease so individuals can be made whole and healthy.

# Table of Contents

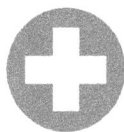

CHAPTER 1

# My Story From Sickness to Health

> *I realized that I wasn't the only one out there experiencing this level of misery. There was a whole community of patients experiencing similar exhaustive, life altering struggles who all needed a miracle*

There was only one answer, self amputation bi-laterally of my legs. I needed to stay alive for my family, so killing myself was not an option, but the pain in my legs was too much. It had to stop. I was a surgeon, I could just cut them off myself. If my legs were gone then the pain had to go away too. My legs hurt so badly that I began to seriously contemplate submerging them in ice water and sawing them both off. My brain was screaming at me to try to find a way to stop the pain and nothing short of amputating them seemed to provide a possible solution.

Logically, I knew that this was not the right answer, but when the pain in your brain is screaming so loudly that you can't hear your own thoughts, you fantasize about any possible solution to ending that pain. At my lowest point, I would not have hesitated to remove them if I knew that it meant that the intense pain that had overtaken my legs and my life would stop for good.

Every day for months, my routine had been the same, I would wake up and try to function in extreme pain while hiding behind a mask that all was well so no one could see what was truly going on. I was a doctor, an OB/GYN. I delivered babies, did complex surgeries, and dealt with other people in extreme pain on a daily basis. Surely, I could get through this. After all, I had a wife and six beautiful children at home depending on me.

However, this wasn't the type of acute pain that ends with the reward of a precious baby birthed into your arms, nor was it the post-surgery pain that although severe at first, gradually tapers off over time. This pain began in my lower back and shot down my legs as if someone had placed searing-hot irons in my bones while my skin felt as if it were riddled with shards of glass. Each step that I took felt like a marathon run on shattered bones and standing felt as if my lower extremities were on fire.

For months the pain had been increasing but determined to continue with my work, I tried to survive it as best as I could. What many people don't know is that just to be in constant pain itself is exhausting. It wears you down physically, emotionally, mentally, and eventually, it will scream for attention so loudly that you won't be able to ignore it anymore.

For me, that watershed moment in my pain journey came at the end of a gynecological surgery that I was performing. Throughout the day, my pain level had been building up and increased with each case that I worked. As I stood during an hour-long surgery the pain began to crescendo until I woke up on the floor, having blacked out presumably from the pain or possibly from a secondary cause to whatever was fighting it within my body. My surgical staff was shocked and attended to me while also safely closing up the patient.

What happened that day changed the trajectory of my life in more ways than I could have ever imagined. I was put on short term medical disability from the University of Kentucky where I was a faculty member and was sent to find answers to the physical pain in my legs that had been plaguing me for so long.

As a doctor, you might think that I would get special treatment while a patient, but I assure you that this is incorrect. In this process, I became a patient just like anyone else, but it is also where I learned some of the most frustrating, yet invaluable lessons.

Some of you have been through the exact same steps that they put me through: first the standard blood panels (CBC and CMP) that revealed nothing, then tests for Rheumatoid Arthritis that revealed low levels of positive RA factor which was then factored out, pain prescriptions to mask all of the symptoms, and when in doubt...injections. When the injections failed, they recommended bulging disc surgery which I refused because I knew that not only were these mild issues, but that at any given time if given an x-ray people can have bulging or slipped discs in many areas of their spine without ever knowing and they rarely cause significant pain. I knew this to be the case with myself.

I had struggled with depression for much of my life, but the physical pain that I was in each day poured powerful waves of depression and hopelessness over me. The doctors prescribed Cymbalta as it dually helps with depression and pain, yet I still couldn't imagine living every day of my life in such a severe state of agony. If it hadn't been for my wife and children, I don't know that I would have been able to keep moving forward day after day. Even while taking five powerful medications and series after series of injections that did not seem to help, the pain was so severe that it made life each day seem unbearable. It was then that I began to fantasize about just removing my legs myself. If I couldn't end my life then maybe I could just end the cause of the pain.

I'm sure that to a lot of you this sounds extreme, but to those of you who have been where I was and have reached that level of pain, you understand it because you have felt it. I'm sorry that you have gone or are going through this, but as awful as it was and as much as I wish that I had never had to feel that level of sustained pain, what I learned from my experience was that God needed to teach me something and sometimes he uses fire to refine us.

As I sat just like any other patient in waiting room after waiting room, I grew increasingly frustrated. I would spend thirty to forty-five minutes waiting for a doctor who would spend one-third of that time listening to me. The doctor would evaluate me, try to treat my symptoms such as my pain, and if no immediate answer could be found, I would either be told to return in several months or passed onto the next specialist. Over the next several months I saw a series of doctors and felt more like a case file and less like person who happened to be a patient. I left one family practitioner to go to one who I thought might be more understanding, then an internist, a psychiatrist, neurosurgeons, neurologists, spinal surgeons, an immunologist, an infectious disease specialist, and after a while I felt as if I was just being passed from doctor to doctor. They knew something was wrong but no one had a solution. Therefore it was easier to make it someone else's problem. Historically, in traditional medicine, this is usually the point where they determine that either it is all in the patient's head or they diagnose it as being a lifelong or chronic condition with no hope for the future except for palliative care in the form of drugs. As a patient, I would have no choice, but to accept the diagnosis, but as a physician, I decided I had no choice except to do everything in my power to prove either diagnosis wrong.

Meanwhile, the pain would have left me bedridden had it not been for my innate stubbornness and desire to push myself to learn something new every day. When you are in constant pain, your life becomes pain centric in that you can not stop yourself from thinking about pain and therefore my quest to learn something new daily became about how to heal myself.

With my brain clouded by medication and my focus torn by the extreme pain burning throughout my legs, I refused to accept this as my new normal and I was determined to regain my life for the sake of my family. Daily, I repeated the excruciating process of dragging myself from my bed and studying to try to find answers. It was through this process that I realized that I wasn't the only one out there experiencing this level of misery. There was a whole community of patients experiencing similar exhaustive, life-altering struggles who all needed a miracle. I was one man drowning in a sea of many who were as desperate to survive as I was. So, as much as possible, I utilized my temporary disability time to study.

While the pain from my legs had overtaken most of the attention of my brain, I knew that there had been other symptoms prior to the symptoms in my legs. These seemed separate, but I did not want to rule out any possible correlation or connection. At the age of sixteen, I had been diagnosed with what was then referred to as regional enteritis, now commonly known as Crohn's disease, and I had been effectively treating this through my diet for years. However, in the months before my legs began their horrific pain, I began to have horrible bouts of diarrhea as well as symptoms consistent with both fibromyalgia and chronic fatigue syndrome (CFS).

For some reason, my body was breaking down and I needed to find the cause quickly before I lost the ability to do so.

Amazingly, my nightmare turned out to be a blessing in disguise. Through my research, I discovered amazing advances that the field of integrative medicine was making at a rate far faster than the traditional medical field. As I started researching this field, the first thing that I noticed was that there was a wide variety of tests available that were not accessible to me or my colleagues that had been treating me in the field of traditional medicine. This intrigued me as I had just been put through the very standard paces of traditional testing and quickly run out of options. To discover that there was a whole field of yet unexplored options out there was something that gave me great hope.

Hope quickly gave rise to a greater interest in this field and a desire to see what potential it had, not only to offer help to me but also others like me. I devoted all the focus that I could muster into studying integrative medicine and the solutions that it offered. This lead to me to discover my own healing, but also inspired me to become a new brand of doctor.

I realized through my research that I essentially had an issue with detoxifying my body and while I began to heal myself through the use of various supplements and treatments, I was able to return to work. However, my eyes had been open to a new avenue of medicine and I was preparing to move forward in this medical field. As I continued working and healing my own body, I also worked to become board certified in integrative medicine. I believed that I needed to have the knowledge and full credentials required prior to starting to practice in the field, unlike some doctors who might claim knowledge, yet lacked the educational backing.

Once my training was complete, my family and I moved to Florida where today I am pleased to provide Crozier Clinic to my patients as a place of hope, so that they never have to experience what I went through, feeling like just a file being passed from physician to physician in the traditional medical system. Here, they can experience the one on one care and personalized attention that every patient longs for and deserves as I partner to pray with them, provide precise answers through individualized DNA testing, and find the root of the problem instead of just trying to mask the symptoms.

Many of you may not be familiar with integrative medicine and how it can help and heal you, which is why I have written this book. I understand what it is like to suffer from chronic pain and to feel marginalized, ignored, or be told that it must be "all in your head." I firmly believe that God has used my own experiences to make me a better doctor and that if you are reading this then He wants you to know that there is hope for you too. God has made the human body in magnificent ways and through integrative medicine, we get the privilege and delight of seeing what occurs when our body is viewed as a whole, these parts can work together to promote and stimulate amazing healing processes throughout.

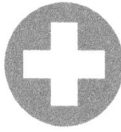

# CHAPTER 2

# Cellular Health: How healing your cells could save your life

*In my own journey from sickness to healing, being able to take a look at what was occurring at a cellular level played a huge part in the discovering a way to heal myself.*

When I first visit with my patients about cellular health, the very mention of this topic sometimes seems to activate an automatic boredom switch. Often patients don't understand or are not interested in my explanations of how good cellular health allows our cells to function, reproduce, and communicate with other cells properly. I explain how each cell in our body is dependent upon other cells to do their job, how the breakdown of cells in one part of the body can wreak havoc on cells in other parts of the body, and that this domino effect of bad cells is what makes people sick. Unfortunately, we live in a toxic world and the natural mechanisms designed to ensure cell health have been damaged. High-stress lifestyles, processed foods, tick bites, chemicals in personal care products, and excessive use of prescription drugs bombard our cells and make it difficult for these tiny, yet essential parts of our total health to perform properly.

In my own journey from sickness to healing, being able to take a look at what was occurring at a cellular level played a huge part in the understanding of what was going on in my own body and the process of discovering a way to heal myself. This, in turn, helped me to find new answers and progressive ways to heal my patients.

I've learned that instead of giving my patients long-winded and complex medical explanations as to why they might be sick and how to find healing, they are better served to hear examples as to how other patients of mine found better health and healing through restoration of cellular health. This inspires them to better understand and follow my treatment plans. I want to share some of these stories with you too. One such story is about a patient named, *Mary*\*.

At sixteen years old, Mary was your typical high school student. She loved running, spending time with her friends, singing in the school choir, was involved in her church's youth group, and took honors and advanced placement (AP) level classes. Her sophomore year of high school, she began having infrequent migraines as diagnosed by her pediatrician--usually just three or four per year. These occurrences were often accompanied by nausea and vomiting, extreme sensitivity to light and sound, and sometimes it felt as if one side of her head was going to explode. These migraines typically occurred only after incidents of very little sleep and therefore were avoidable if she avoided fun things like sleepovers with her girl friends. However, occasionally even those fun experiences were worth justifying the payback of an awful migraine. If she did happen to get one then she would just hide away in her dark, quiet bedroom and sleep until the pain and sickness subsided. Usually, she didn't even need

---

\* All patient names are pseudonyms in order to protect their privacy.

basic over-the-counter medication to help. She just needed her two younger siblings to stay mercifully quiet for a few hours.

Once Mary graduated from college, she earned a collegiate scholarship for running cross country. Her migraines seemed to subside as she maintained a very disciplined training, dietary, and sleep schedule. For almost four years she seemed to be migraine free as she maintained the life of a typical college student with grades that earned her a spot on the Dean's List each semester. She also participated in long hikes up the local mountains in Eastern Kentucky, occasional boyfriends, and sometimes weekend parties.

One week, Mary's joints started aching all over and she was so tired that she slept through practice. This was the first practice she had ever missed in her four years running for the University. Her coach was so worried about her that he personally came by after practice to check on her. When he found out from her roommate that Mary was sick, he insisted that she be taken to the physicians at the campus health clinic. There she was told that she had a 104.3-degree fever and most likely a nonspecific virus and was given instructions to rest, drink fluids, and told that she would most likely recover within 5-7 days.

Mary's fever did subside, but the fatigue and joint pain remained. She also had frequent terrible headaches while she had been sick and was worried that the migraines of her teen years were back. Her coach suggested that maybe easing back into practice and regular movement would help with both her fatigue and joint pain. He said that he had heard that some other students on campus had a similar virus, so Mary tried not to let the fact that her whole body felt as if she were running through quicksand each practice bother her. Her headaches went away, but in swirled a brain fog that rarely lifted. She couldn't concentrate in class and she couldn't even make it through a full-length practice anymore, because her muscles felt too fatigued and her joints and bones ached as if she was framed in shards of glass. Her coach sent her back to the clinic, who sent her to the hospital to run some blood tests. The blood tests indicated a generally high level of inflammation but didn't test for anything specific so the clinic once again attributed it to the viral infection that she had previously been ill with.

Mary struggled through her senior year of school, finishing what was supposed to be her pinnacle year as a runner unable to make qualifying times. Her fatigue and pain overwhelmed her to the point that she would miss classes and when she did attend, she felt as if her brain was too fuzzy or foggy to retain the information. As a result, she barely passed courses that she would have aced prior to this.

When her parents visited her at graduation, they were shocked by her physical appearance. As a long-distance runner, she had always been lean, yet well-muscled. Now, she appeared emaciated. Instead of her usual strong, powerful gait, she hobbled slowly forward, clearly wracked by pain, eyes sunken and lifeless. Her family immediately arranged to take her home, canceling her summer internship and instead arranging for her treatment. Initially worried that perhaps she was suffering from anorexia nervosa, they spoke with her coach and found out what had transpired as Mary hadn't been forthright with them; not wanting to worry them.

They first took her to a Primary Care Provider (PCP) who spent ten minutes with her, ordered some labs, and asked her about the pressure of the last semester of school. He did find out about the virus but thought that the joint pain was probably not related. Once finding out that she was a runner, he asked if most of the pain seemed to be located in her legs. Mary hesitatingly answered yes, as throughout the years her ankles, knees, and hips had seen their fair share of tendonitis or other running-related overuse injuries. He then prescribed her medication that in theory helped with both joint pain and depression as he felt that she was simply suffering from end of the year stress coupled with old joint injuries. He felt that this medication could treat both. He also prescribed her narcotic for use if the pain became overwhelming. He told her that he would look over the labs and see her back for a follow up in a month's time.

One month later, Mary returned to the doctor with her mother. This time, the visit was seven minutes long. The labs were normal except for high levels of inflammation which could be indicative of virtually anything. Mary and her mom were both in tears reporting that the medications had not helped except for the narcotic which offered only small bursts of relief and she was using as often as possible. The doctor decided to increase Mary's dosage of both medications, the first of which he explained should help not only her joint pain, but also what appeared now to be the possibility of depression as both she and her mother stated that she barely moved out of bed. In addition to re-prescribing the narcotic in a larger amount, he also prescribed an extended release version of an opiod, a painkilling medicine that could now be active in her body all day instead of at increments like the narcotic. This way she could still use the narcotic on an as needed basis, theoretically lessening her chance of addiction to it's narcotic properties. They were to follow up in three months.

Three months later, Mary returned to the doctor unsure of whether or not the medication was truly helping, yet too scared to stop it and possibly causing another increased amount of pain. She had gained thirty-seven pounds since beginning the medication for depression and joint pain, and was no longer underweight but was in fact slightly overweight for her height. Her joints still ached over her entire body, but her PCP seemed very focused on her leg joints--given her young age, her relatively good health, and her athletic history, so he decided to send her to an orthopedic surgeon for an evaluation.

Mary waited six months for the orthopedic surgeon to evaluate her, order x-rays, and then tell her what she already knew. That her hip, knee, and ankle joints had the beginning of some tendonitis and perhaps even some arthritis. However, this time Mary's father interjected, "what does that have to do with the overall joint pain she is experiencing?" The doctor seemed unsure but ordered an MRI of her lower back, pelvis, and all her lower extremities. Her dad had mumbled something about how expensive this was getting despite no conclusive results being found. Then the doctor prescribed her an additional medication for joint pain.

Mary was now on four very powerful medicines with no solid diagnosis. So far her only medication side effect had seemed to be the thirty-seven pound weight gain from the depression/joint pain medication, but the newest prescription for joint pain changed this. In three months, Mary gained fifteen more pounds. Her parents also noticed she exhibited extreme anxiety about doing typical things that she used to enjoy. She no longer wanted to leave the house, go out in public, and started having regular panic attacks accompanied by restlessness and erratic behavior. They didn't initially attribute this to the medication, and instead assumed that she was self-conscious about her weight or struggled from depression related to dealing with the pain. While those are definitely factors that may have contributed to her depression, the sudden changes in behavior signaled side effects from the medication.

Meanwhile, Mary was distraught, she felt like her entire life had fallen apart and she hated every bit of her new normal. It had been nearly two years since she had gotten sick with the "virus" at school and now the orthopedic surgeon was recommending surgery on both of her knees which he had eventually decided must be the source of the problem. Mary would have done the surgery if she thought it would have made the pain stop, but her parents felt as if that couldn't suddenly be the problem. Meanwhile, Mary's PCP had become convinced that it was fibromyalgia and prescribed three times daily doses of medication for fibromyalgia.

Then Mary's headaches started again. Could her migraines have come back? They didn't feel the same as her migraines from high school. She now had these every single day for six months. They were different than before. They were mostly in her forehead and down the back of her neck. They didn't make her sick, but they were still miserable, all day, every day. Her doctor tried a daily medication, then added an additional medicine, known as an abortive, to stop the migraines once they started. When this failed, he tried another combination of the two types of medications plus he added a course of thirty-one botox injections into her head and neck muscles every twelve weeks. She underwent this process several times and it failed several times. She was exhausted and felt ready to give up on life. Her parents were drained but were not willing to give up on her. Her siblings were weary and felt the strain of their parents' time, energy, and finances all going towards one child as they continued the parade from doctor to doctor in search of an answer.

Thankfully, for a patient like Mary, there is hope in the field of Integrative Medicine. However, it is unfortunate for Mary that she wasn't able to see me first and skip the endless carousel of traditional medical doctors. These doctors, in trying to treat her symptoms and not her cellular health, were only making her worse.

As I shared in my own healing story, my medical practice was transformed and I helped patients just like Mary gain healing through the practices of regenerative, genetic, and cellular therapies. I've witnessed miraculous results and transformed the lives of my patients which is why they come to see me from all over the world.

Cells are the microscopic building blocks of the human body and when these blocks are damaged or destroyed, this is where illness and breakdown happens. Through the marvelous and exciting process of discovering the damaged cells and regenerating them into stronger cells, we can gradually see the healing and restoration process begin.

For a patient like Mary, I can't help but wish that she had come to me at the beginning of her health struggles. Her traditional medical doctors responded much like I would have when I was in the traditional medical field and the way that we were trained to in medical school...to quickly treat the symptoms with prescription drugs developed by "approved" government bureaucrats at the Food and Drug Administration (FDA). However, much like her physicians, I would have been unintentionally harming Mary without ever getting to the root of her problem.

Now, as an integrative medicine physician, who knows that the integrity of the cellular structure determines the health of your body, the first thing that I would have done is listened to Mary's entire story and evaluated her on a cellular level. While being attentive to Mary's story, I would have discovered that her main symptoms were initially fatigue, joint pain, and fever. I would have also noted that she had migraines as a teen that seemed to be well managed. I would have learned that she was a cross-country runner in Kentucky and during her training, she would have often gone through grassy areas, woods, or locations of high grass or weeds. She also loved to hike which would have further exposed her to similar areas. She had no known tick bite with rash but said that the runners often pulled ticks off their socks and once she found one in her hair. She had a fever for less than a week, but the joint pain and fatigue remained. After two years on high levels of medication, she also had a sudden surge of daily migraines. Fatigue, joint pain, and even headaches can be indicative of many things, therefore it is not hard to see why these symptoms may have been improperly diagnosed even if a doctor spends an hour or more with each patient as I do.

However, this is the critical aspect that I believe would have saved Mary so much time and agony--I would have diagnosed Mary through the use of genetic testing from the very beginning just as I do with all of my patients. To have the knowledge of Mary's cells and her DNA at the outset of these problems could have prevented her and her family so much pain and hardship. Together, we would have been able to assess her cellular makeup and therefore immediately diagnose and treat her as having Lyme disease, which is in fact what she had.

Instead, she did not receive the correct treatment and the issue lingered for years and would now be considered chronic Lyme disease which is more difficult to treat. She had been on eight different types of very powerful medications with varying side effects that instead of helping her were actually adding to her symptoms and increasing her side effects. For example, the pain medications that she had been given and been taking for years with increases over time were causing "rebound headaches" also known as "medication overuse headaches." Due to these headaches, she would take more medication which would have increased the pain and headache cycle putting it into a never-ending overdrive. The second medication that she was placed on for joint pain had not helped her at all and in fact, had only agitated her mental state. Thankfully, her parents eventually noticed that specific drug's harmful side effects and were able to talk to her physician about their concerns and remove her from it before it caused lasting damage such as suicide.

This is why I can not emphasize enough, the importance of building your body's health on a strong foundation by looking toward revolutionary integrative, regenerative, genetic, and cellular therapies that can literally harness the power of your own cells in order to create functional tissues. These cells rebuild tissue walls and repair bodily organs that have been damaged due to age, disease, or congenital defects. Isn't it amazing that God made your own cells with the capability to access, restore, and repair damaged areas renewing functionality to the body and healing us one cell at a time?

This is also why I am surprised that when people say that I am revolutionary for being perhaps one of the first doctors worldwide to check the DNA of all of my patients and that there are still only a handful of physicians are doing this. This is a practice that can save lives and prevent the development of diseases and illnesses like Mary's long before they gain the momentum to destroy lives. The earlier a problem is found and the sooner that it is treated, the better the outcome tends to be for the patient.

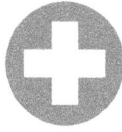

# CHAPTER 3

# Traditional Medicine: Limitations for patients

*Integrative medicine combines the best principles and practices from other types of medical studies such as traditional medicine, regenerative medicine, and even functional medicine.*

When discussing integrative vs. traditional medicine, I find that most people have a very full understanding of traditional medicine as would be natural given that they have experienced it most of their lives, but their knowledge of integrative medicine is limited. Until my new normal in life lead to radical change and healing, this was my experience too. I knew everything there was to know about how traditional medicine functioned. After all, I was a physician, but I found that through my experiences with both illness and pain, traditional medicine was very limiting. Thankfully, I was introduced to integrative medicine at the time in my life when I most desperately needed more answers and more options than traditional medicine could give. As I was blessed to be able to gain healing from it, I would like more patients to experience the benefits of integrative medicine on their paths to wellness.

Traditional medicine is simply what the name suggests: medicine based on an extensive history and tradition involving patients presenting with symptoms while doctors seek to provide a diagnosis followed by a treatment in a linear fashion. The

World Health Organization (WHO)[1] defines it as "the sum total of the knowledge, skill, and practices based on the theories, beliefs, and experiences... used in the maintenance of health as well as in the prevention, diagnosis, improvement or treatment of physical and mental illness."

It is this system of medical treatment that we are most used to in the United States. Patients get sick, they go to the doctor, and they expect to be sent out the door with a treatment that fixes whatever ails them. However, due in part to government regulations, greed from insurance companies, a broken medical model, and its inability to treat the person as a whole; traditional medicine is failing.

How is it possible that what has worked traditionally for so long, could be failing now? As the medical structure changes and continues to be insurance and monetarily based, physicians are rapidly becoming disillusioned within a few years of entering the workforce.

Physicians who got into medicine because they cared about people are rapidly retiring or quitting to pursue other careers. Due in part to the Electronic Health Records mandate of 2009, time spent doing paperwork has increased while time spent between physician and patient time has decreased. The average primary care physician has two-thousand patients and three-fourths of physicians are suffering

---

1   https://www.who.int/traditional-complementary-integrative-medicine/about/en/

burn out.[2] Physicians who thought they were getting into a business of patient care, instead found that they were becoming highly educated secretarial staff which was not what they had trained for nor envisioned for their careers or futures.

Currently, the insurance companies are controlling the costs for the medical world and have the ability to approve what tests a patient may or may not be allowed. With the high premiums the insurance companies charge, they should work for the patient and not the other way around. This can be an increasingly frustrating problem especially as you seek treatments that the insurance companies choose not to recognize in order to save themselves money. For example, in the early two-thousands, the insurance companies denied the existence of chronic Lyme disease in order to avoid paying for the treatment of it. Thousands of patients suffered, growing sicker and remaining undiagnosed because in large part the insurance companies simply didn't want to have to pay for the testing or the subsequent treatment. This is unacceptable.

Physicians are increasingly put under pressure to see more patients due to doctor shortages and insurance companies wanting higher profits. Currently, the average amount of time that doctors spend with patients has decreased to thirteen

---

2  https://www.forbes.com/sites/sallypipes/2018/10/15/government-policies-are-driving-doctors-to-quit-health-care/#6012389c2bf3

minutes.[3] That is average. It is often less. In less than thirteen minutes, how is a doctor supposed to adequately address and diagnose the physical needs or otherwise of a patient? We are asking doctors in the traditional medicine system to do the impossible and yet, it seems as if nothing is going to change anytime soon. This is the system that has the insurance and infrastructure support behind it to continue taking money and treating symptoms instead of people.

Doctors are constantly pressured to treat the symptoms. Often the fastest way to address a particular symptom is to write a prescription that helps to temporarily stop or relieve that symptom. As this doesn't look at the individual beyond the solution to the symptom, it often just masks the problem, causing side effects that then appear to be other symptoms that eventually need treatment. The patient deteriorates and the original root of the problem is never found. Due to this, I firmly believe that the traditional medical community is making patients sicker. If you don't diagnose the reason for the problem, then how can you heal the patient? You can not. Blindly prescribing medications in the hope that one of them works is akin to playing Russian roulette with your patient's health.

I myself was part of this failing system of traditional medicine, both as a doctor and as a

---

3   https://www.statista.com/statistics/250219/us-physicians-opinion-about-their-compensation/

patient. Don't get me wrong, I am not opposed to traditional medicine, although the current system needs an overhaul. I believe that the medical community can do better and that is where the use of integrative medicine comes in.

Early in my career as a physician, I was just like many other doctors who saw a revolving door of patients. Spending time hearing each of their health stories didn't seem a luxury that I could afford, so they cycled in and out and I treated them with kindness, but not with the time that was truly needed or deserved.

Then, my own illness turned my life upside down in a way that I never expected and gave me a "new normal" in which I had to learn how to start life over. As you already know, that changed my approach to medicine forever.

As a traditional doctor, let's say I had a patient *Heidi*, who came to see me as an OB/GYN complaining of anxiety, depression, insomnia, and trouble "connecting with her husband." Heidi was forty-five years old and therefore after a short visit with her, my training would have taught me that the most likely option was that she was in perimenopause and I would have ordered tests in accordance with that and tried to give her symptomatic relief by perhaps prescribing a sleep aid and/or anti-depressant while also recommending a lubricant to help aid with any possible vaginal dryness, etc. associated with the symptoms of perimenopause.

The amount of time that I would have been able to spend with her would have been greatly limited, so my focus would have been based on her symptoms and not her life circumstances. If the prescriptions treated her symptoms and she was able to gain some relief then she would have most likely been at least satisfied enough with her treatment not to return until something else gave her other or additional symptoms and I would have felt that my job as a doctor had been completed.

Meanwhile, while I would have been patting myself on the back for a job well done, Heidi, left that same appointment feeling discouraged and upset. She was hurt and embarrassed that a doctor would assume that she had vaginal dryness when that was not the case and in her mind, I ruined her trust and lost all credibility. She also didn't agree that she was in perimenopause as her menstrual cycle had always been like clockwork, there were no hot flashes, night sweats, or any of the other symptoms that her mother or older friends used to complain about with menopause. She most likely would not get her prescriptions filled, because she now didn't trust my judgment and was left feeling more depressed than before. In addition, she would now feel even more ashamed to open up and ask for help. Doctors in the traditional medical field are letting patients like Heidi down all the time in the search to treat symptoms instead of heal patients.

This traditional style of treatment was fine with me until I experienced it as a patient and spent more time in waiting rooms then interacting with my doctors. Then I myself got frustrated being viewed as a list of symptoms instead of a person who had an underlying condition that was causing these symptoms. I was tired of doctors trying to find a quick fix and prescribe medications that masked or made me sicker instead of getting to the root of the problem. I saw first hand how traditional medicine was failing our patients as it was failing me. It was then that I decided to make a huge change. I transitioned into the practice of integrative medicine.

Integrative medicine combines the best principles and practices from other types of medical studies such as traditional medicine, regenerative medicine, and even functional medicine. Integrative medicine will merge the western medicine that most of us have been ingrained with while adding a holistic or whole-body approach. This will allow us to continue to treat patients with an understanding that each part of the body works in coordination with other parts and systems and therefore the individual must be viewed as a whole in order for proper diagnosis and treatment. As medicine continues to develop, so does the need for integration of various treatments and techniques that address the body as a whole. I believe that we need a well-rounded arsenal of approaches to get to the root of the problem, not just throw a medication or supplement at a symptom.

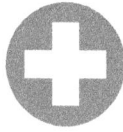

# CHAPTER 4

# Integrative Medicine: Healing at the root

*My new normal has taught me to view each of my patients through the eyes of not only a physician, but also as someone who has suffered through sickness and a never-ending parade of doctors.*

Now that I practice integrative medicine, the process for diagnosis and treatment is a whole different ball game. What is integrative medicine? Integrative medicine is a type of medicine that prioritizes the patient placing them in a partnership with their physician as they work together to establish a personalized health care plan that treats the individual in their entirety and not just their symptoms.

Therefore in my practice, this means that I sit down with each patient and talk with them about all aspects of their health--physical, emotional, environmental, social, mental, and spiritual. I believe that God created all parts of our being to work together in harmony and that it is important to address and treat our body as a whole and not just focus on a certain symptom that might be masking a much larger problem underneath.

There were so many times that as a patient that I felt ignored, unheard, and that is one of the reasons that I love the partnership of integrative medicine. It means that your doctor becomes your teammate and you work together to face and fight your health issues instead of feeling as if your physician is your foe. In integrative medicine, the physician becomes your best advocate and you are not alone in championing to find the best solution to a healthier and healed you.

As an integrative physician, if the patient Heidi, from the previous chapter came to visit me and expressed the exact same symptoms (anxiety, depression, and insomnia), not only would I sit and listen to her to get a fuller and more complete history and understanding of her life, but I would also have a genetic test done to get to the very core of the problem. This eliminates any guesswork on my part and narrows things down very specifically to tell me what exactly needs to be treated. In Heidi's case, I discover that she, in fact, is not experiencing the early phases of menopause, but instead has been grappling with depression after the loss of her mother, combined with the daily stresses of being the primary caretaker of her two young children while her husband's job often takes him on the road. If it weren't for the time I was able to spend with her, the doctor-patient relationship built, and the combination of DNA results along with other labs, then the root of her problem would have continued to go unaddressed and untreated. However, through my proven method and the power of integrative medicine, Heidi and I were able to work out a specific plan suited just for her and I am happy to report that she is feeling better than she has in years. Praise the Lord!

Often, patients that have struggled for years with chronic illness or unexplained symptoms are frustrated and disillusioned with the current medical system. Like me, they may have sought out "the best of the best" in the medical community only to be given no answers, shuffled off to other doctors, or told, "it's all in your head." To someone that is suffering, this is a devastating outcome and to have it happen repeatedly, is to lose hope over and over until you are left with none.

As someone who used to be clinical faculty at a University medical facility, I realized that we have a flaw in how we are training our medical practitioners. We are training them to be excellent linear thinkers, but poor critical thinkers. Linear thinkers work well in a traditional medical setting wherein a patient comes in with a specific set of symptoms, they will order the corresponding set of labs, and the predictable medications. Seems simple right? It could be unless you are a patient who presents with abnormal symptoms. This type of patient requires a critical thinker to diagnose them. In other words, someone who thinks outside of the box. On the popular television show, *House, MD.*, Dr. Gregory House was a brilliant example of a critical thinker. His character, modeled after the great literary detective Sherlock Holmes, did not stick within the conventional bounds of linear thought, but examined all potential possibilities and aspects of a person's life that could possibly contribute to their health and wellness. Although, I am certainly not suggesting that any doctor behave like the fictional Dr. House, the ability to critically think when assessing a patient is crucial in helping them find healing. Every patient is as unique as their DNA and therefore, their conditions often present completely differently. As a result, sometimes a medical-style Sherlock Holmes investigation is exactly what is needed and integrative medicine gives me the freedom to pursue the case of each patient until the answers are found and the case is solved restoring a sense of hope.

This is why it is so important to me to spend so much time with my patients today. My new normal has taught me to view each of my patients through the eyes of not only a physician, but also as someone who has suffered through sickness and a never-ending parade of doctors. I can truly listen with compassion and empathy. Although difficult to go through, I believe that God has used my sickness as a tool to bless and help others in ways that I could have never imagined--listening to my patients is only the beginning point. The number one characteristic that is attributed to Jesus in the Bible is compassion and in wanting to walk in His example, it is essential that I exhibit and that my patients feel my compassion for them through our work together.

Through integrative medicine, I can then partner with them to make an evidence-based plan that specifically suits their needs and their genetic types.

We are able to use the body's own God-given healing mechanisms to promote more natural and less invasive recovery. Integrative medicine is based on great science but is always open to the idea that there is constantly more to discover and learn, so advances are being made every day. This is exciting news for my patients because it simply means that there are new answers being continuously found and as your partner in this process I am always looking for a solution to help improve your personal health.

It is my belief that we need to get to the heart of the problem and develop a personalized, well-rounded treatment plan. If at all possible we need to find the root cause of the problem, then we need to consider the role that genetics plays in each individual case, determine what function of the body is exhibiting dysfunction, and finally evaluate what the best modalities are for restoring normal function to the cells, organ systems, and overall body.

Once we have done all these things, we can develop an individualized plan for your health. I get increasingly upset with current treatments because they are protocols verse catered patient care. The problem with protocols is that they take a one size fits all approach without taking into account that we are all individuals with different DNA and different biological pathways that need care or correcting. Therefore one treatment doesn't fit all. I deeply feel that we need individualized care for every patient.

Let's partner the science with the individual. Integrative medicine allows me to work to suit your specific needs and create a plan that is just right for your body. I know that your body can be restored because my own body was restored. I was told that it was impossible, yet with God all things are possible. Through my own experiences with integrative medicine, I was able to heal myself and I believe that I can help do the same for you. Don't give up!

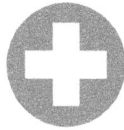

# CHAPTER 5

# Genetic Testing: Why and how to test your genetics

> *Your DNA is very much like a biological instruction manual that explains what shapes you, how you were formed, and can even predict future illness.*

I believe that God designed each human being, perfectly and intricately in a way like no other. Therefore, it makes sense that our genetic code would reflect the wonder of our creation in our greatly varying DNA patterns. This is also where I believe that medicine cannot take a one size fits all approach. Just as our bodies are uniquely made, so are our reactions to the environment that we live in.

While searching to piece together the sum of all the chronic illness symptoms that had been plaguing me for years and finally narrowing it down to a specified known cause, Lyme disease; I wholly devoted myself and all my time, energy, and resources into beating this disease which had been trying for so long to beat me. In studying my patients with Lyme--whether those with confirmed tick bites or those with similar symptoms, I did something that no one else in the world was doing at that time. I took DNA samples from each patient in order to try to evaluate the root cause from a cellular level. This allowed me to study the DNA of Lyme patients more thoroughly through comparing and contrasting a broad range of samples. More importantly, it gave me the ability to make treatment plans that catered specifically to each individual and their precise genetic make-up.

Currently, in my practice and with patients around the world, I continue to stay ahead of the curve through the use of a revolutionary new genetics-based health care program, called *Gen1:1*, designed to help you understand how your genes influence your health. I believe that God created us each with our own unique genetic code or DNA, which is why I call the program *Gen 1:1*. Your DNA is very much like a biological instruction manual that explains what shapes you, how you were formed, and can even predict future illness.

We all have different allergies, sensitivities, and reactions to the world around us and it is through studying your genetic makeup that we can identify potentially harmful genes and can then form a treatment plan that caters directly to you and your individual DNA profile. God created all of us as unique as the human fingerprint and in doing so, physicians like myself are advocating that individuals need individualized care instead of the opposite.

For those suffering from chronic conditions, social media has become an invaluable tool for patients to seek others struggling with similar conditions to form and participate in groups where information can be collected, shared, and exchanged. This can provide an amazing opportunity for people to connect with those who are sharing similar health struggles. One thing

I often find in examining these groups is that in addition to the important community support aspect found, is that often people ask their fellow group members whether or not a certain medication will cause side effects. They might get hundreds of varying and contradicting responses: "yes, that medication gave me significant hair loss." "No hair loss here, but how about the weight gain?" "I lost 75 pounds and my migraines are now gone too, totally worth it." "The weight gain is awful, but I actually stopped due to the blindness." "How do you like those hallucinations?" "No side effects whatsoever for me…, etc."

How can one medication affect so many people completely differently when they all have been diagnosed with the exact same condition? The answer is of course that their DNA is thoroughly different, so their prescribing doctor is simply playing a game of trial and error to rule out what medication works and what does not, in regards to their condition. However, with DNA, we can target precisely and eliminate all the guesswork. What other benefits does treating your health through genetic testing have for you? Here are a few:

1. You can reduce the risk of certain diseases and potential health scares.

2. Make efforts to prevent disease to help you live a longer life.

3. Adjust dosages of and/or avoid certain

medications to increase safety and decrease certain side effects.

4. Help you understand what foods to eat, what to avoid, and what is most beneficial for your body.

5. Reduce symptoms from current illnesses.

6. Help you to live a more full and abundant life with the illnesses that you already have.

How does this testing work? Similar to a DNA kit that you might order to tell you about your family heritage, this test gives us a wealth of information on your health heritage and potential wellness future. Simple to use, this test can be delivered to your house where it requires only a saliva sample. No blood test required! Then it is shipped to the lab for your DNA to be analyzed and the results to be evaluated.

I will review your personal results and develop a treatment plan that is right for you based on your unique genetic health care risks. You will be amazed at what you can learn through this simple test and how precisely and specially God created each aspect of your genetic design. Through this plan you will learn how to: prevent disease, detoxify your body, and live life to the fullest.

Let's take my patient *Magnus* for example. A few years ago, Magnus, a middle-age man and good friend of mine; came to see me to feel better, increase his energy levels, and live a healthier life. I was happy to help him out. Along with speaking with him about his health concerns, he was evaluated through our genetic testing program. Some patients are nervous to see these results, fearing that they will be sent pages of endless numbers that they can't decipher. This is not at all the case. The report that each patient receives explains everything in a very detailed, yet simplified way with careful instructions on how to avoid health pitfalls and plans to live your healthiest life. Additionally, I add my own notes to emphasize what I think is most important for you to know throughout the report. No need for concern, I do not have the typical illegible handwriting associated with most doctors.

In Magnus' report, we discover what the best "matching diet" would be beneficial for him in order to maximize gene expression as well as identify what diseases he was most at risk for if he didn't change his current lifestyle. This means that the report shows what particular dietary recommendations work best for his specific body type. Since we aren't all genetically the same, not all diets work the same for each individual. The misconception that there is a one size fits all approach to dieting causes discouragement and frustration which is something that we want to avoid and is one reason that I believe your dietary plan needs to be specifically suited to you. In Magnus' case, it is important for his genotype to be on a low-carbohydrate diet. Interestingly enough, it also reveals that he has an enhanced bitter taste perception and therefore may not favor certain bitter-tasting vegetables. Isn't it fascinating that from his DNA, we can tell that Magnus most likely does not take his coffee black?

In addition to finding out what diet type would best suit him, we also discover that his genetics leave him at high risk for arterial hardening, high blood pressure, stroke, and heart disease. In order to combat this he will need to increase omega-6 and omega-3's in his diet as well as supplementing these vital fatty acids as well as consuming both vitamin B1 and B2. He will have to be extremely vigilant given all these factors as far as his diet goes to combat the potential of heart disease, but thankfully due to the very specific map of his DNA, we know exactly what foods he should take and what he should avoid to create the perfect path to wellness for him.

Magnus' genetics also indicate a low level of folic acid in his blood and a need to supplement it. This directly correlates with his vitamin B deficiencies. If Magnus were a woman, then we would pay extra attention to the need for folate in his diet during his child-bearing years. Potentially this could cause neural tube defects or have other devastating side effects for a pregnant mother and child and to counteract this she would be instructed to take supplements such as prenatal vitamins with an increase in folic acid if there were any chance of becoming pregnant.

Two fascinating sidenotes, his entire life, Magnus has felt a never-ending hunger. He could snack all day and still be hungry, or eat a large meal and still want more. While in his youth this may not have made much of a difference, as he ages, this can dramatically affect his weight and health. It turns out that genetics has an explanation for this. He has a genetic variance called NMB which means that he literally feels hungry more often than the average person. Being cognizant of this will help him to better manage it in the future to avoid overeating.

The second side note of interest is that Magnus discovers that he has a rare gene found in short distance runners/sprinters. When he was younger he, in fact, had run the 50-100 yard dash in track and field, confirming this interesting genetic find. Even as he aged, he found that for fun he could use this genetic trait to his advantage to challenge the younger, cockier boys to short races that utilized quick, small bursts of speed and still come out ahead. I don't want to embarrass him, but there is a rumor going around that he pulls out this trick at parties and tries to make money by getting people to bet against him. Lesson learned...don't accept his bet. Even his genetics back this up.

Through his genetic tests, we are able to help get Magnus on a healthy dietary plan for life. One that best suits his body's genetic needs and helps keep the potential risk for heart disease at bay. We are able to supplement precisely where needed and encourage the increase of foods that naturally contain those supplements. This is not a temporary diet or short term change. This becomes his new way of wellness--a healthy, healing, and restorative life just as God intended it to be.

It is God's desire that all of us live life to our fullest potential so that we can glorify Him with the gifts that He gave us. I know this seems an insurmountable thing to do when it is a struggle just to live life daily with chronic conditions. It is my desire to use the tools that God has given me to help you in your own journey toward reclaiming your life and living abundantly in Christ.

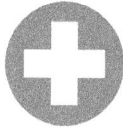

# CHAPTER 6

# Nutrition and Genetics: Eat more of what your body needs, less of what it doesn't need

*In studying the genetic makeup of each of my patients, I have learned how important it is that our bodies have the correct nutrients to help create an environment that promotes and stimulates healing.*

While growing up, a healthy diet was something that was always emphasized in my family. My mother set this example for my family by baking bread for us each day, preparing healthy meals with fresh ingredients including vegetables from our own garden, and even encouraging the use of vitamins and dietary supplements. As someone who has suffered from Crohn's disease since the age of sixteen, I quickly learned that maintaining a healthy diet was important to maintaining my own wellness in relation to that disease. However, it wasn't until I began to delve deeper into the study of integrative medicine and the effect that nutrients played on our genetics, that I realized how important it was that our bodies have not just healthy nutrients, but to have the correct healthy nutrients to stimulate genetic healing and proper gene expression.

As I continue to see physicians in the field of integrative and regenerative medicine use advanced healing methods to benefit their patients, I have noticed that there is a portion of patients that are not being benefited by these therapies and I believe that I have isolated the reason why. In studying the genetic makeup of each of my patients, I have learned just how absolutely important it is that our

.ıe correct nutrients in them to help
. environment that promotes and stimulates
.ııg. As most physicians only undergo four hours
.ıf nutritional education within medical school, this
is absolutely one way in which most physicians are
failing their patients. A correct diet is the fuel that
keeps the body running at peak capacity and if we
aren't providing our bodies with the right fuel then
it is doomed to breakdown and failure.

My desire to learn more about this and how I
could use people's genetics to change their health
was sparked through the meeting of a specific
patient named, *Brianna*. Brianna was initially in a
wheelchair, devastated by genetic disease. She had
started undergoing cellular treatments and was
making dietary changes. Miraculously, I was able to
witness her life change completely as she went from
being wheelchair-bound to standing, then walking,
and regaining her life again. It was so inspiring to
see God's healing hand and I knew that I wanted to
be able to help maximize people's cellular treatments
to their greatest effect and I believe that as with
Brianna, proper specialized nutrition is the key.

Long before there was ever "big pharma," God
gave us an abundance of plants, animals, fruits,
trees, herbs, and it tells us in Genesis one that He
"saw that it was good." Now, I am not saying that
I think that medications are bad or should not be
used, because I do think that they are important
at specific times and for specific jobs. However, I
think that God did a wonderful job of creating the

nutrients that we need to help maximize our health and healing.

Many of my colleagues have written books with protocols for changing your diet and healing the symptoms of your disease and a lot of these highly respected physicians were originally banned from the medical community for introducing these ideas. However, after years of proving that food can indeed work as medicine, these physicians' voices are finally being heard and respected again in the medical community.

Although I agree with the food as medicine thought process and the emphasis on a correct diet, I get very upset with the current protocol treatments as they are essentially cookbook diets and do not take into account that everyone's body responds differently to a certain assigned diet or protocol. The problem with protocols is that we are all individuals with different DNA and different biological pathways, therefore one treatment does not fit all. Science gives us the ability to exactly match what each person needs through the evaluation of their DNA, so why wouldn't we use that information to maximize the health and well being of each of our patients?

Imagine your body was a highly tuned race car, would you go to the gas station on the corner and put some regular unleaded gasoline into it? No, you wouldn't dream of it, yet that is what we do almost every day. Our bodies are magnificent works of our

They can be used liberally in place of salt or artificial flavoring.

7. Moderation is the key.

Be aware that your body is unique and no one else is made exactly like you, which is why it is so important to cater to the needs of your body's specific DNA nutritional needs. Your best friend may lose weight existing on an all protein and high fat diet, but not only is this not sustainable nor heart healthy for a lifetime, it may be the exact wrong thing for your genotype. You may try it and it may cause nothing but frustration and ill health. This is why it is so important to meet with someone who understands your body's genetics thoroughly. Together, we can specifically guide you away from the choices that can have lasting harmful effects on you, and toward the things that can change your life forever as you take steps to join me in creating your healthy future.

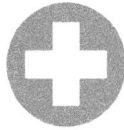

# CHAPTER 7

# Gastrointestinal Dysfunction and The Brain: Your brain-gut connection

> *Both the brain and the gut play such an integral part of the immune system that if one of them is not working correctly we will lack a complete immune system.*

Now that you have spent several chapters learning about a variety of subjects, before we delve into our study of the gut, it is time for a short quiz to test your knowledge on the etymology or source of the name of this very official-sounding term *gut* when used in the modern medical field in reference to the body's digestive tract.

What is the originating source of the term *gut* as used in today's modern medical field?

    a) The term *gut* was first published in a 1957 paper on the digestive system and its effects on immune health by Scottish Surgeon Dr. James M. MacKenzie and British Dr. Frank W. Randall as they felt it was a better descriptor than it's Latin counterpart.

    b) Gut is a shortened term for "gullet to buttocks" which describes the entire digestive tract from entry to exit.

    c) Old English word used as early as/or prior to the 14th century for bowels or entrails.

    d) All of the above

Congratulations! You have finished the quiz and as your prize for winning you get the coveted "bragging rights" and if you got it wrong then you get to learn something new. The only truly correct answer is C, so if you answered C then you win bragging rights which I'm told that at least in the 5th and 6th grade boys sector of life is a really huge thing. If you got it wrong then don't worry, no one will ever know unless you circled your answer with an ink pen in which case, I guess you are out of luck.

There is really no explanation for how gut became such a common descriptor even in the medical community except for the fact that it is a simple way of describing something that everyone understands so easily, which is that the gut makes up the digestive system, also known by the more official-sounding name, the enteric nervous system (ENS). The enteric nervous system or gut works in direct relationship with the central nervous system (CNS) which is made up of the brain and the spinal cord. These two systems must maintain a proper balance in order for the body to function correctly.

As someone who has suffered with Crohn's disease from childhood, which wreaked havoc on my digestive system and bowels, as well as suffering neurological conditions including Bell's palsy in relationship to Lyme disease, it would have been very easy to completely separate the conditions and claim that they were so different as to not be connected to each other. However, that is not how God created our bodies. He uniquely created each part of us to work together as part of a system that creates the whole being of who we are. Therefore, we can not underestimate the power of the brain-body connection nor its overall connection with our immune system.

As a medical student, due to my own complex medical history...not just with the pain in my legs, but also having Lyme disease since second grade and Crohn's disease since the age of sixteen, it became especially important for me to understand how the gut was interconnected with both the neurological and immune systems. While working as a physician assistant in neurosurgery, neurology, and ophthalmology; I began to see how the brain affected every organ system in the body. It is important to see how the brain and body work together to regulate the various systems to keep everything regulated. The brain controls many bodily functions working through nerve fibers, neurotransmitters, and hormones to try to bring homeostasis (balance) throughout the body.

The primary function of our intestinal tract is to digest foods, this begins in our mouth with saliva starting the first enzymatic breakdown of food elements. As the food breaks down, it continues into our intestinal tract where the pancreatic enzymes enter the small intestinal tract and aid in digestion. Then good nutrients are transferred across the mucosal lining into our blood system and taken to various organs and throughout the body for the distribution of needed nutrients while the unneeded particles are eliminated through bowel movements.

In our gut, we have special cells that help produce an immune response. Their role is to protect the body's immunity and defend it against all sorts of pathogens. They basically act as protective soldiers in our body's immunological defense by setting of an inflammatory signal when a bacteria being transferred across the intestinal mucosa alerts them that something is wrong. Both the brain and the gut play such an integral part of the immune system that if one of them is not working correctly we will lack a complete immune system.

If these cells respond to unsafe bacteria in the system they can trigger an immune response causing inflammatory issues. Acute inflammatory issues are usually sudden and short-lasting which is different than the continuous, chronic inflammatory issues which can eventually lead to inflammatory bowel disease.

Bowel disease is also known to be associated with other neurological complaints such as depression. Growing up, I experienced both of these issues. As a child, I experienced severe abdominal pain for years with no solid diagnosis. Depression accompanied this sickness to the point that in 6th grade, I began an attempt to take my life by hanging myself in the shower that was interrupted by my mother. A few years later, depression would once again lead to an attempt on my life that thankfully the Lord saved me from so that thankfully I can save the lives of others.

Depression is a widespread problem in the United States as well as throughout the world and it continues to be on the rise. Although depression can be situational, as previously shown--the brain and the body are so highly interconnected, that it would be neglectful not to explore every possible avenue that ties the issue of depression with overall health and well being. As we know how clearly the ENS and the CNS are related, it is therefore highly possible that depression is rooted in the gut and not just in the brain as most people assume. I believe that we are doing a disservice to those struggling with mental illness or mental health issues when we don't assess the body as a whole and work to correct the gut and digestive issues that can wreak havoc on our brains as well. A holistic approach needs to be emphasized when we approach this issue.

For example, in individuals suffering with depression, there is usually a lack or loss of serotonin, the good feeling that chemical nerve cells produce. As scientists identified this loss of serotonin in the brain, this brought about the advent of the classification of drugs called selective serotonin reuptake inhibitors (SSRIs). These medications work by increasing the level of serotonin in the brain and decreasing the reabsorption of it back into the brain which in theory would produce or make more happy chemicals in the brain. However, what if the problem is actually the creation of serotonin and once again we are treating one symptom without focusing on the body as a whole?

probiotics, health was restored and the teen began to gain a healthy amount of weight. The mother was ecstatic because after years of frustration and watching her child go through one difficult procedure after another, the answer had been found. Ian, who had been struggling with a large amount of depression along with their illness, not only saw physical healing, but mental healing as well and was soon back in school, happy, and driving around just like a typical teenager. The depression had been diagnosed as mental illness and treated as such, but when we found the root cause was in the gut we were able to wean him off antidepressants and instead treat him effectively through his diet. This yielded nearly immediate positive results, yet without any negative side effects. This is the type of result that a physician desires for all of their patients and is indeed the result that I desire for you.

On the flip side, we are far behind on our understanding of the brain's effect on the gut. This began a larger search for understanding the gut's effects on the brain and the brain's effect on the gut especially in reference to the conditions of attention deficit disorder (ADD), attention-deficit/hyperactivity disorder (ADHD), and some conditions on the autism spectrum. There are two main camps of theory on these issues in regards to the brain-gut connection or vice-versa in combination with gene expression.

The first would obviously be similar to what we just discussed in regards to depression--the gut has some issues affecting homeostasis in the body and disrupts the connection between the ENS and CNS causing the brain to not work entirely correctly. Theoretically, you fix the issue in the gut and this helps to heal the issue. For example, a child with ADD might really be struggling with a gut issue but instead be treated with medication aimed at symptoms that affect their brain. While these medications might appear to work, they may also have huge negative side effects, changing the child's inherent personality and dulling their mind while never actually healing the problem, especially if the problem is indeed a gut issue to begin with.

Another theory that few people like to address is that as our small children go about their daily lives, they receive small concussions in secondary daily play or sports activities. Think about how many times a toddler bumps their head running into, well...everything. These small concussions could have a large effect on the gastrointestinal system. They can decrease motility of the GI tract and when motility is slowed in the GI tract we develop abnormal microbiomes. This then leads to a progression of problems including the neuroimmune connection, but also other factors may be associated with these concussions such as ADD, ADHD, learning disabilities, as well as possible psychological issues. Although, this is a very possible theory, for me it is the most unlikely of either as the brain is very forgiving when young and is still changing and growing.

The third component that I believe contributes to these issues is gene expression and plays a part either way. I believe that all of the aforementioned conditions have a genetic component and that is where gene expression and activation comes into play.

It is very important that we continue to study these issues to determine where the reaction was first, in the brain or the gut; yet know that as we look to heal the problem we must evaluate the problem as a whole and treat the parts as one.

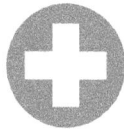

# CHAPTER 8

# Gastrointestinal Dysfunction and GI Health: How to heal your gut

> *In starting the healing process for the gut-brain immune system, I believe the number one thing that we must do is to take control of our thoughts and our thought life.*

Increased intestinal permeability or what some refer to as "leaky gut" is a disgusting sounding yet commonly used term for a process that can actually be quite typical in our body's GI system. It actually refers to the permeability of the mucosal layer and the gastrointestinal system.

In simpler terms, our GI system is made to be permeable, allowing nutrients to be taken out into the red blood cells and distributed throughout the body. Serotonin is distributed in this same manner. At the proper levels of permeability, the cell junctions of the gut remain tight and the mucosal layer does not allow any toxins to pass into the bloodstream. This is important because the gut is the largest immune system organ in the body.

The system needs to be at the perfect balance of permeability to let the nutrients out into the bloodstream while keeping the toxins, waste, and undigested food particles moving towards excretion.

We already know that there is an increased intestinal permeability plays a role in Crohn's disease, irritable bowel syndrome (IBS), and celiac disease with some studies showing that it may be associated with other autoimmune diseases, although the evidence from clinical studies has still yet to be seen.

Like most fathers, for me, one of the hardest things in the world is to see a child suffering, and when my daughter developed a painful, weeping rash that made her extremely self-conscious, I wanted to find answers for her. We took her to a series of physicians, pediatricians, and gastrointestinal specialists who seemed to think that it may be food-related, but couldn't provide a solid diagnosis nor relief. Meanwhile, my daughter was suffering from the pain of her rash, but also was constantly trying to hide it as she was embarrassed by its appearance. Finally, I decided to investigate on my own. The only causative agent that I found in her system was a protein called zonulin.

Zonulin is a protein, discovered by Dr. Alessio Fasano in 2000, that changed the way that doctors and scientists viewed bowel permeability and was truly a novel and breakthrough discovery. As we now know the gut is made to allow nutrients into the bloodstream, but keep toxins and waste products out. However, in what was termed leaky gut there seemed to be a breakdown in these usually tight junctions that was somehow allowing toxins to get into the bloodstream and potentially contribute to all manner of autoimmune responses. When the protein zonulin was discovered, it was as if the key to unlocking these tight barrier junctions had been found. The zonulin protein had the ability to cause great amounts of damage by squeezing itself into these tight cell junctions, essentially regulating them by forming gaps that allowed toxins to then freely flow through the newly created gaps that the zonulin proteins opened. This discovery introduced a whole new aspect of bowel permeability. It was as if these zonulin protein blocks were acting as little door holders to allow toxins or other particles to freely flow out of the gut into the rest of the body spreading their toxicity and causing illness or breakdown.

Zonulin affects digestion, absorption, hydration of the body, homeostasis, and the trafficking of environmental toxins across the mucosal lining of our very delicate gastrointestinal system. Many individuals tested negative for celiac disease yet were still were having unbelievable amounts of similar symptoms such diarrhea, constipation, bloating, skin rashes and irritations, fatigue, canker sores, poor weight gain, unexplained behavioral changes, and unexplained weight loss ended up testing positive for the zonulin protein. Therefore, it is surprising to me that more labs are not able to do routine testing for zonulin as it has been nearly 20 years since it's discovery. Thankfully, in my own lab, this is something that I easily have the ability to test for.

We must make sure that all of our nutritional needs are appropriate so that we can regulate the Zonulin protein molecule. We know from some studies that increasing fermented foods may help in the alteration and production of this protein molecule. Any foods that cause inflammatory responses in our body also cause an increase in zonulin and therefore should be avoided. Increasing our fiber intake also helps to modulate the production of zonulin as fiber helps with elimination and the assurance of proper probiotics in our digestive tract. If we keep these factors well regulated then we should be able to maintain low levels of zonulin in our body and maintain a healthy gut and therefore improve our overall body health.

Going "gluten free" and advertising foods with "no gluten" has definitely been the trend of the last decade or so, but with the exception of those with celiac disease or a true gluten allergy the real problem could actually be a substance called carrageenan. Carrageenan is an extract derived from red and purple seaweed and is commonly used as an emulsifier or thickening agent in a variety of foods including everything from yogurts, breads, deli meats, nut-based milks, ice creams, cottage cheese, cream, chocolate milk, baby formula, and a variety of vegan based products. Touted as "all-natural," people assume it's safety while forgetting that many all-natural substances...for example tobacco, can have deadly side effects.

The problem with carrageenan is that it is extremely inflammatory to the bowel and has been closely linked with not only inflammation, but also with bloating, IBS, glucose intolerance, colon cancer, and food intolerance. It is, however, the inflammatory response that causes an alteration and increase in zonulin levels. Figuring out the root of your child's problem or your own could be found by eliminating this one destructive product from your diet or could save you from potential problems in the future.

There was a young boy named *Roger* that cried non-stop for the first two years of his life even when he was held and soothed by his parents around the clock. He had not had a solid night's sleep in two years and neither had they. As an infant, they thought that he had an extreme case of colic combined with acid reflux. He had been given formula since birth and the pediatrician thought there could potentially be an allergy, so he was rotated through one expensive formula after another with no change in symptoms. He was given a battery of tests and examinations that revealed nothing. He started doing repetitive "stim" type behaviors and some doctors theorized that maybe he had autism. His poor parents would ask for volunteers just to hold him as he cried so they could get some rest, sleep, or time with their other children.

By the time I heard Roger's story, he was two years old and had been eating solid foods for over a year and had inconclusively been diagnosed with a myriad of possible bowel problems or food intolerances. However, he was still struggling. He was still stimming, was verbally and developmentally behind, cried nonstop, and barely ate, yet maintained an almost bloated appearance.

Through DNA testing, it was identified that he had a severe inflammatory reaction to carrageenan which had been in his diet since he began taking formula as an infant. Once his diet was properly adjusted to suit his DNA and carrageenan was eliminated, Roger, became a different child. He stopped crying, quickly caught up in his speech and motor skills, and his stimming ceased completely. It was discovered that both the stimming and crying was due to the fact that this poor baby was just trying to cope with being in constant pain. This sweet family was given a fresh start due to some dietary changes that altered and reduced inflammation and corrected his gene expression. They were so relieved once their little guy started to sleep and became a truly different child. They felt guilty that they hadn't sought out DNA testing earlier, but they simply hadn't known it was an option and in truth should never have felt guilty as they were doing the absolute best with the knowledge that they had. I am often seen as the last resort doctor when traditional medical options have been worn out, but this is the opposite of how things should be. If more patients pursued integrative doctors as their first line of defense, they would save a lot of time, money, and despair.

If you are sick and you know that you have a neurological, gastrointestinal, or immunological problem, I would advise that you find a healthcare practitioner that will look for the root of the problem and not just prescribed a medication for the symptoms. Finding these individuals may be difficult but be persistent. I also want to encourage you to be patient, because just as it takes time for healing to occur, you did not get sick overnight and it was most likely a gradual breakdown that occurred over a long period of time. Believe that you get will get well, follow directions from your physician, and you will improve.

In starting the healing process for the gut-brain immune system, I believe the number one thing that we must do is to take control of our thoughts and our thought life. The word of God states that we must take every thought captive to make it obedient to Christ (2 Corinthians 10:5) It is evident that through our thought life we begin to speak life or death. (Proverbs 18:21) Due to the fact that the power of life and death is in the tongue, we need to control what is coming out or our life. Positive thoughts bring positive words. God spoke things into existence and we are created in His image, therefore, we need to speak health into existence.

Our bodies are the Temple of the Holy Spirit (1 Corinthians 6:19). We are instructed to take care of our bodies and in doing so we must be diligent to take in proper nutrients and make sure that nothing vile comes out. As in Hosea 4:6, we can no longer say that we are a people dying from lack of knowledge because as a population today we are well informed with an abundance of knowledge.

We have been given knowledge about foods, water, healthy air, and more, but the difficult aspect is disciplining ourselves to eat correctly and drinking what is healthy for our bodies, avoiding contaminated foods. There are forty-nine scriptures in the Bible on self-discipline. I believe that the large number of scriptures on this topic only further emphasizes its importance. We also think that the need for self-discipline applies just to being overweight or over-eating and it certainly does as being overweight increases your inflammation levels and puts you at higher risk for many chronic diseases and illnesses. However, self-discipline is important for all aspects of life and dietary management as it takes a tremendous amount of discipline and training to make significant or even small changes to our long term diet.

One of my favorite scripture on self-discipline is 1 Corinthians 9:24-27(ESV) *"Do you not know that in a race all the runners run, but only one receives the prize? So run that you may obtain it. Every athlete exercises self control in all things....But I discipline my body and keep it under control, lest after preaching to others I myself should be disqualified."*

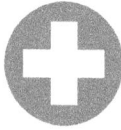

# CHAPTER 9

# Lyme Disease: The silent culprit behind many diseases

> *Lyme can masquerade. If you don't know or understand the root cause, then you may spend a lifetime suffering from and fighting Lyme symptoms that will only worsen over time.*

As an eight-year-old child, I had been bitten by a tick while playing in the Minnesota woods near my home. At this time, I was an intelligent, adventurous, active second grader with a zest for life and fun. Following the tick bite, I became increasingly sick, bedridden, and eventually lost the ability to read. I had always been a bright young boy, but with the loss of my ability to read came other learning challenges including a dyslexia diagnosis and I went from the top of my class to not being able to pass my grade. My parents took me to multiple physicians, but no one ever even asked my mother about a tick bite and I certainly wasn't tested for Lyme disease. For years, I struggled with physical ailments with no known root cause. My journey with Lyme is documented in detail in my book, *Ticked Off*, but suffice it to say, Lyme altered my entire life. Discovering that Lyme was the root cause of many of the problems that I struggled with...the immense pain in my legs, fibromyalgia, chronic fatigue, Bell's palsy, depression and more, spurred me to learn as much as I could about the disease, making me a foremost expert in the field. With over 300,000 new cases of Lyme disease being diagnosed annually, it is difficult to believe that so many physicians still deny Lyme as a diagnosis. It is estimated that there were are over 100,000 patients annually presenting with Lyme symptoms put through the gauntlet of practitioners: physicians, physician assistants, nurse practitioners, specialists, and naturopathic doctors only to be misdiagnosed and unvalidated as someone struggling with Lyme disease. We need to do better as a medical community.

Practitioners who take their time to evaluate for Borrelia burgdorferi or Lyme disease, become suddenly aware of the very dangerous effects of Lyme and how frequently it actually occurs. Some physicians refer to it as the "great masquerader" or "great imitator" as it frequently mimics other diseases. This makes it more difficult to diagnose and therefore is a disease that often goes untreated.

Most individuals with Lyme disease do not remember a tick bite or in the case that they do, can't recall ever having an associated "bull's eye rash." This rash is one of the key indicators that practitioners are trained to look for in regards to Lyme, so its absence can cause confusion. This missing element in the chain of diagnosis can be critical as Lyme is primarily known as a tick-borne illness. I do not want to sound like an alarmist, but there are now studies linking it with other vector-borne transmissions including mosquitos. As it is an illness transmitted through the bloodstream, we need to be open to the possibility of varying transmission methods. Worldwide there have been increasing amounts of articles and studies linking Lyme to transmission through other forms including mosquitoes, mites, flies, and more. It is encouraging to see other countries studying this disease as it is definitely not just a North American problem.

As the spirochetes identified in Lyme are very similar to the spirochetes also long identified in syphilis, scientists are continuing to test the theory that Lyme could be sexually transmitted as well. This, along with the possibility that Lyme could be passed through the bloodstream and therefore be present in donated blood could have huge implications on the future of many people and therefore need continued investigation and study.

It is frustrating to discover that there are many physicians throughout the country that Lyme does not exist in certain states. This is a false assumption. Others believe that all Lyme began and was transmitted from a centralized location near Lyme, Connecticut and related conspiracy theories abound. Although this location is where significant groupings of cases were first brought to attention in the US, this is also a false supposition. In fact, in 2012, when scientists did a work-up of the 5,300-year-old cro-magnon "Iceman" found in the Eastern Alps, it was shown that his genetic analysis revealed Lyme disease. It is discouraging that with all we now know about Lyme, practitioners still commonly tell their patients that they can not have Lyme as they don't believe that it is present in their state. This does a disservice to the patient in delaying an accurate diagnosis and presenting them with a false sense of security. Often this stops patients from pursuing Lyme as a diagnosis and they grow sicker because of it. Unfortunately, I do know that the majority of physicians read few articles outside of their specialty outside of their residency which leads to a deficit of knowledge and mistakes in diagnoses.

We saw through Mary's diagnosis at the beginning of this book just how easily Lyme can go undiagnosed, yet how important it is to get a correct diagnosis from the beginning before a chronic condition develops. Knowledge is power and therefore arming yourself with all the knowledge necessary to identify and therefore fight against this disease is of the utmost importance.

I think that it is important that I inform you of the symptoms of Lyme, so that as a patient you can be educated, allowing for less of a chance of a missed diagnosis. The following are symptoms or associated conditions of Lyme disease and are also outlined in my book, *Ticked Off*:

- The presentation of a"bullseye rash." As I stated before, this does not occur in every individual, but when it does, it should be noted. This rash usually begins within three to thirty days after the initial bite. It is important to add that other

insect bites or skin reactions can present with
similar bullseye type rash, so it is important
to have an experienced practitioner closely
evaluate each one. Some reports state that in
only twenty percent of cases of Lyme is there
ever presentation of a rash--this means that
eighty percent of the time, no rash is present.
However, in my practice, only four to six
percent of patients report having a rash with
the remainder exhibiting no rash. Therefore, I
believe that the expectation of the presentation
of the bullseye rash is possibly a weak indicator
for this disease. Even with the presentation
of a textbook bullseye rash, physicians who
deny the presence of Lyme in their state or are
poorly educated about Lyme will misdiagnose
it and cause the illness to go untreated. This
means that if a physician is looking for the rash
as the only indicator of the potential of Lyme,
a concerning amount of patients are going
undiagnosed. Physicians and patients need
to be educated about the prevalence of Lyme
disease and the fact that this telltale rash truly
exhibits very rarely.

- Bell's palsy. Bell's palsy is another often
overlooked, yet serious symptom of Lyme.
Twice as a teenager, I experienced this
phenomenon, with no known explanation at
the time. It typically presents with muscular
weakness causing one half of the face to

obviously droop. Once while I performing with a traveling music team in front of a crowd, I was embarrassed to have a sudden, significant droop to my face. This disappeared eventually, only to re-occur at a different time in my life. It wasn't until I began my study of Lyme that I was able to connect the two. Bell's palsy can be missed by a large number of practitioners who do not realize that this is a very common symptom of Lyme disease. Many individuals simply have not looked through medical literature showing possibilities and indications for Bell's palsy and there is plenty of misinformation mistaken for common knowledge. This is a prime example of physicians clinging to old, or outdated knowledge without the study of newer data and possibilities. Many patients are told that Bell's palsy is a self-limiting problem that will go away. This is not the case as self-limiting would indicate that there is no root cause. The droop may possibly disappear but that does not mean that the root cause does not remain. Early detection of this may help prevent the neuroborreliosis (the neurological symptoms) inflicted by Lyme disease.

- Excessive or chronic fatigue. Fatigue, in general, is an extremely common condition, affecting more than seventy-six percent of individuals diagnosed with either Lyme or other disease processes. Fatigue is so prevalent that it can often be very difficult to find a root cause for this debilitating symptom. Often associated first with causes such as stress, high workload, sleep apnea, or viral sources such as mononucleosis or Epstein-Barr, this symptom can be difficult to diagnose. In fact, ninety-nine percent of patients that I've seen in the past that present with chronic fatigue also have had elevated Epstein-Barr levels, so perhaps these symptoms and this virus go hand-in-hand. Fatigue is a symptom that is often ignored or generalized as few truly understand the difference between simply feeling tired, verses true overwhelming and unrelenting fatigue. Although Epstein-Barr may not actually be a symptom of Lyme, chronic Lyme can cause immune dysfunction, activating this already commonly occurring virus and thus resulting in devastating fatigue. Therefore, fatigue of this magnitude must be carefully paid attention to and the possibility of its connection to Lyme, seriously considered. In the case of fatigue that is diagnosed as myalgic encephalomyelitis/ Chronic fatigue syndrome (ME/CFS), this condition in itself is disabling as a person can experience never-ending fatigue that is not improved by rest or any amount of sleep. As physicians, we need to do better in finding the root cause of diseases such as this and be aware that there is usually an underlying culprit.

- Night sweats. Night sweats are a very common symptom of Lyme, but can also be symptomatic of other diseases or conditions and therefore needs to be carefully evaluated.

- Fibromyalgia. Fibromyalgia is often closely tied with chronic fatigue, occurring simultaneously, and therefore we commonly find it associated with Lyme. However, by nature fibromyalgia causes significant widespread pain due to overactive nerve endings. This causes unbelievable muscular nerve pain which can result in insomnia and fatigue which could be the primary relation with fatigue, or it could be Lyme associated. However, I should note that the majority of the time fibromyalgia is identified, I've been able to identify mold as the culprit.

- Cognitive impairment. This is a common complaint of Lyme patients due to the fact that neuroborreliosis, or the neurological manifestation of Lyme disease, will impair neurotransmitter receptor sites and release endo and exotoxins, resulting in significant mental decline. Other chronic conditions, such as fibromyalgia, contain symptoms of "brain fog" or memory loss, so it is once again important that the root cause is found.

- Arthritis. Arthritis was one of the first things noted among the grouping of children in diagnosed in the late seventies and early eighties in Lyme, Connecticut. These arthritic pains can be extremely intense and initially, individuals were often diagnosed with rheumatoid arthritis. When in the case that samples are collected from an aspiration from the inflamed joints, the telltale Lyme spirochetes are often noted in many of the individuals with arthritic complaints. If the practitioners are not looking for Lyme, they can give a simple diagnosis of rheumatoid arthritis while missing Lyme as the underlying causative agent.

- ALS. ALS or Lou Gehrig's disease is a very devastating diagnosis. Not everyone with ALS has Lyme. However, out of the few patients that I've treated with ALS over half of them tested positive for borrelia recurrentis, a genus of the spirochete phylum bacteria which is vector borne and known to cause relapsing fever. This is a different bacterium than Borrelia burgdorferi which is most often associated with Lyme, but it is one of the thirty species of borrelia. Patients diagnosed with ALS and far enough advanced in their condition that they have lost their ability to walk have undergone treatment with me and been healed, regaining the ability to walk and other lost functions. One outcome is a slow, terrible decline towards death while the other indicates healing. I continue to witness patients that once treated successfully report back to their big name hospital institutions exhibiting evidence of healing to be met with a lack of enthusiasm by their practitioner or a lack of desire for that practitioner to know how they could help their patients recover in this same manner. Instead of curiosity and a humble desire to learn about how healing was accomplished, they haughtily remain in ignorance. I find it continually disappointing when the medical community cannot work together to accept out of the box thinking or is reluctant to embrace new treatment methods. Universities are performing their own studies, but not sharing any of the knowledge gained from these studies and this is detrimental to the community as a whole.

- Depression and psychological problems. As you have seen from my own story and my struggles with depression and suicidal ideations, depression can be a real entity with Lyme disease. Psychological changes also are a part integrated with neuroborreliosis, which are the neurological manifestations associated with Lyme disease. Shockingly, it is estimated that medical conditions causing mental health issues affect as many as twenty-five percent of psychiatric patients. We can not overlook physical causes in mental cases. In one published article in the *Journal of Psychiatry*, thirty-three percent of the psychiatric patients showed signs of Borrelia burgdorferi antibodies also known as the antibodies used to fight off the Lyme causing bacterium[4]. Many patients who have targeted Lyme in their treatment have completely reversed their neuropsychiatric behaviors. I have witnessed this personally with my own patients. Some of the psychiatric disorders seen in Lyme patients include: memory impairment, dyslexia, seizures, anxiety, panic disorders and attacks, psychosis, violent behavior, rage, mood swings, sleep disorders, ADD, ADHD, obsessive-compulsive disorders, and depression.

- Autoimmune diseases. I believe the exact cause of autoimmune diseases is poorly understood. We do know that autoimmune diseases are a response of our own body essentially attacking itself. Above we discussed that one such disease, rheumatoid arthritis is often associated with Lyme and the possibility that Lyme is in fact, the causative agent. There are other autoimmune diseases that have been associated with Lyme disease. It is estimated that approximately forty-five percent of those

---

4   https://ajp.psychiatryonline.org/doi/full/10.1176/appi.ajp.159.2.297

suffering from Lyme also have Hashimoto's thyroiditis. Therefore, we can see it is not just associated with autoimmune arthritic conditions, but with other autoimmune conditions as well. Although not everyone with an autoimmune disease has Lyme, I believe that Lyme can be a genetic stressor of sorts that causes incorrect gene expression, resulting in the development of these autoimmune disorders. For example, we may have genetic markers that already predispose us to certain autoimmune diseases, but these are in some way activated when placed under an additional stressor such as Lyme disease. I know that my experience with genetics may cause me to differ from a lot of other physicians in observing that this may possibly be helpful, but I like to combine all aspects of the tools at my disposal to see the totality of the individual in order to aid them to total body health. For instance, some individuals with specific genes can predispose individuals to autoimmune diseases and our knowledge of this could help more quickly identify this or work to promote healthy gene expression, potentially avoiding these conditions. Although it is not yet clear, scientific research seems to indicate that genetics combined with certain external elements can cause certain genetic autoimmune based reactions. Changes in lifestyle such as diet, removal of environmental toxins and biotoxins, and other significant actions could prevent the expression of these autoimmune disorders altogether.

In reading through this list of symptoms, you might identify several that you yourself struggle with. You may have been diagnosed with other unrelated conditions not associated with Lyme and it is indeed possible that Lyme is unrelated to what you are experiencing. However, as Lyme masks itself in some extremely common symptoms, it makes the most sense that if you have any of these symptoms to rule Lyme out as a diagnosis. If Lyme is at the root of what you are fighting, wouldn't it be best to know this? If you don't know or understand the root cause then you may spend a lifetime suffering from and fighting symptoms that will only worsen over time. I know from my own, personal experience that this only causes pain and devastation. We need to identify the root cause in order to work to fix it. In discovering healing at the root, the related symptoms will be healed as well.

Physicians need to be responsible to push to find healing solutions, but patients also need to remember to not settle in finding solutions for optimal health. Patients can help challenge physicians to find new solutions by advocating for answers and not accepting less than the best care. In turn, physicians need to challenge themselves to never stop learning and growing in their fields. If they open their eyes to continued to study and education, this will benefit their patients and their practices.

As notable figures such as celebrities are open about their struggles with illnesses such as Lyme, it increases the platform for knowledge as well as funding in this field. As people continue to push and advocate, advances will be made. Hopefully, this will be the future for Lyme.

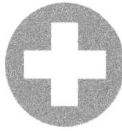

# CHAPTER 10

# Stem Cell Therapy: The new frontier of medicine

*Stem cells unique ability to adapt in order to regenerate into various cells allows a qualified physician like myself to place live, healthy stem cells precisely where they are needed in the body to stimulate cell repair replication and restoration of cellular function.*

At age seventy-six, golf legend, Jack Nicklaus was in debilitating pain. He had struggled with a lifetime of back pain, but now hitting a golf ball was excruciating and he could not stand for more than ten minutes at a time. That same year, in 2016, he underwent an experimental stem cell therapy in Munich, Germany that allowed him to play golf again.

Using stem cells taken from his own fat tissue and injected directly into the origin of pain, Nicklaus credited the procedure for helping him to become pain-free, return to his golf game, and allowing him to once again stand for unlimited amounts of time. In fact, the procedure was so successful, that he was planning to return to the clinic to have a similar procedure done on his rotator cuff and had referred both his sons to the clinic to undergo the same outpatient stem cell treatment for their own back issues. It had been a life-changing treatment.

Other famous athletes, such as soccer star Cristiano Ronaldo, are also reported to have undergone stem cell treatments for injuries with much success. In his case, for a ruptured hamstring, with all accounts stating that the results were positive leaving his injury site feeling better than it had in the past two years.

As more reports like this pop up in the news, you may have wondered if stem cells might be a solution for you? Patients often wonder if this kind of treatment is only for athletes or would also work for them and their particular condition? As stem cell treatments are still relatively new in the United States, patients often don't know where to begin their search for a physician or what field of study this branch of medicine falls under.

In 1992, Leland Kaiser coined the term "Regenerative Medicine" boldly proclaiming "A new branch of medicine will develop that attempts to change the course of chronic disease and in many instances will regenerate tired and failing organ systems."[5] It may sound like something straight out of a science fiction movie, but regenerative medicine is actually a simple concept to understand, based on the principle of using the human body's naturally existing repair mechanisms. Although regenerative medicine is a relatively new science with continuing and dynamic research, it is solidly based on molecular biology and helping the cells regenerate, restore, and replicate to repair them to normal function.

Described as transactional research, regenerative

---

5   Kaiser LR (1992). "The future of multihospital systems". *Topics in Health Care Financing*.

medicine, strives to use scientific findings and take them from a laboratory or research setting into practical application and patient treatment. Therefore, regenerative medicine's aim is to directly benefit patient health. Why is regenerative medicine important? As scientific discoveries grow by leaps and bounds, this allows my ability to serve you better as a physician to grow by leaps and bounds as well. Therefore, it is critical that you understand at least the basics of this amazing science. Often patients who visit me feel discouraged by prior physicians who have left them feeling bereft of all hope, struggling in the mire of chronic conditions. I know this feeling all too well as it is something that I endured too.  However, once patients understand regenerative medicine at even a basic level and that new breakthroughs are continuing every day, it gives them a reason for optimism and encouragement.

So, simply put, what exactly is regenerative medicine? I think that the average person understands that as far as wound care, the body has a natural tendency to try to self heal. You get a cut or a small wound and your body forms a scab in order to heal it. Now imagine this on a cellular, tissue, or organ level where in some cases, self-healing isn't a possibility and the condition languishes...or would, if not for the intervention of regenerative medicine.

For example, long before it was even termed regenerative medicine, some of the earliest practices in the field were organ transplants. Let's imagine that a heart valve transplant surgery is done. The patient's own heart would have failed without the surgery, so this restores the heart to mostly normal function, however, the heart is already compromised after years of dysfunctional use and the new valve can't hold up as well to the wear and tear of the already compromised heart. This is where the magic of the latest innovation of regenerative medicine comes in and where I begin to get really excited. Instead of using other organs or organ parts to try to help stimulate healing in the body that in the past would eventually fail, we can more effectively do this at an even smaller level with less surgical risks and greater physical rewards through the use of stem cells. We can inject stem cells directly into the weakened organ tissue where they can then replicate, regenerate, and heal.

As patients struggled to find treatment options in a system that had often left them discouraged, passing them from doctor to doctor without answers, or told that their fate would be a lifetime of suffering...which is to say, no life at all; many blazed trails trying more "experimental" options outside the United States and came back with positive experiences and stories of hope. Some of these earlier individuals were wealthier "Celebrity Types" with the money to travel to Europe, South America, Central America, or other countries where medical testing doesn't take nearly as long nor is regulated as safely as it is here in the United States. As they returned and shared their positive stories in various media outlets, other's soon followed suit. However, let me caution you that I have treated several patients who were damaged following supposed stem cell injections outside of the United States. Every year over three-hundred and twenty thousand United States citizens leave the country to pursue alternative healthcare treatment and half of these patients are going internationally for stem cell treatments. Not only is this unnecessary as we are able to do the same treatments here in the United States, but we are able to do it in a way that is regulated and safe. In fact, I am one of less than fifteen hundred physicians in the US injecting stem cells and have trained extensively to do so. Therefore do your research and make sure that wherever you go you are getting live stem cells from an accredited physician.

In the early days of stem cells, celebrities went abroad in search of various treatments in youthful rejuvenation and vitality not yet offered in the United States. They often weren't sure what the exact treatments entailed, just that they yielded favorable results. What they were actually getting was injections of sheep stem cells. Since they were derived from the cells of sheep, they were initially available in more abundance. Injected or dripped intravenously (through IV's), the thought was that they may help provide more energy and perhaps give the skin a more youthful appearance as well. These early treatments greatly underestimated the multifaceted abilities and use of stem cells and hadn't even begun to scratch the surface of what science would begin to unfold as the use of the human stem cell took over and an infinite number of possibilities for healing seemed to open up. In fact, now through the use of human stem cells, there are treatment possibilities for a wide range of problems such as multiple sclerosis, ALS, dementia, Lyme Disease, Parkinson's Disease, visual problems, and a whole host of other conditions with previously very few treatment options other than palliative care.

Let me be clear, I must strongly caution my readers, about the importance of doing your research and finding a trusted physician and accredited facility when seeking these kinds of treatments. As someone who suffers myself from chronic illness, I know the desperation that can be felt in the search to find healing or cessation of pain at almost any cost. While this often opens your mind to possibilities of trying new procedures or experimental science, it simultaneously makes you more vulnerable to potentially dangerous products or situations. Especially when your medical expenses have already drained your financial resources and you are looking to cut corners to cut costs, you are incredibly susceptible to scammers or dangerous practitioners who may be savvy enough to build a professional website but in the meantime their lack of medical expertise could cost you your life. Be incredibly wary and cautious about making plans to travel abroad for treatment. I always emphasize that you can never be sure what products you are getting and it could potentially be dangerous, so please be sure to do you due your due diligence and stay informed. I also must say that no matter what country you are in, it is important to make sure that when using stem cells, your physician is injecting you with only the most healthy cells so that they can effectively regenerate and reproduce. I must emphasize this because I have been appalled to find that some physicians give poor quality or even dead stem cells. This will cause complete failure and is a waste of time and money. Not to mention, further ruining of the fragile relationship of trust between patient and doctor, when the patient may already feel that this is their last resort. As a physician, the safety of my patients is paramount and this is why I always go above and beyond to receive every available accreditation to ensure the safety of my patients.

Whether it was an individual in pursuit of some sort of stem cell fountain of youth or a patient desperate to find the one thing that would finally bring them relief through healing, patients were driving a push to find healing through regenerative medicine options. This patient driven push is what has helped the field of regenerative medicine expand and grow within the United States which now provides patients safe, FDA regulated options that they can pursue within our own country.

In fact, now through the use of human stem cells there are treatment possibilities for a wide range of problems such as multiple sclerosis, ALS, dementia, Lyme Disease, Crohn's disease, autoimmune disorders, Parkinson's disease, osteoarthritis, neuron growth, visual problems such as macular degeneration, and a whole host of other conditions with previously very few treatment options other than palliative care.

A friend of mine refers to stem cells as "nature's pharmacy" and I wholeheartedly agree. These amazing cells are found within our own bodies and enable us to recover from illness and injury in just a fraction of the time when given to patients to help in the healing process.

So what exactly are stem cells and how does this relate to you? Anatomically, the human body is composed on a large scale of eleven major systems such as the skeletal system, nervous system, or respiratory system. On a slightly smaller scale and within these systems are the organs themselves. For example, the cardiovascular system would contain the organ of the heart, respiratory the lungs, and so forth. So far, that seems pretty simple, right? Now, each of these organs is made up of tissues. However, they are not each made up of the same types of tissues and sometimes an organ is even made up of several varying types of tissues. The systems work interdependently, meaning that they must all work together to function, but they all function in a variety of ways and therefore all require specialized tissue best suited for their unique purpose. Therefore, just as a building utilizes a variety of materials for construction, so our bodies also require various tissue types to build our differing organ and system parts.

This is where things literally get microscopic--on the cellular level. It is these microscopic cells that make up your body's tissue. There are many varying types of cells, but most are made to do very specific jobs. For example, most people are very familiar with erythrocytes which are more commonly known as red blood cells. We may not have all seen these cells under a microscope, but we know that their job...their ONE job is to carry oxygen through your body and remove carbon dioxide through your lungs. Many cells are like this, where their purpose is already "differentiated" or chosen at development. Stem cells are special because unlike these differentiated cells they can become or "differentiate" into a vast amount of different types of cells. This allows them to regenerate and then replicate into virtually any type of organ system.

Stem cells' unique ability to adapt in order to regenerate into various cells allows a qualified physician like myself to place live, healthy stem cells precisely where they are needed in the body to stimulate cell repair replication and restoration of cellular function. This makes it possible to regenerate cells once thought impossible to repair. These amazing superpowered stem cells can help restore spinal cord injuries, joint, tendon, ligament, and muscular injuries, and even cartilage damage.

We already know that stem cells are basically cells with super-power abilities, but truly just how powerful are they? I knew a patient who was in need of a lung transplant, yet was quite far down the transplant list and his family knew that it was very possible that he would die never making it to the top of that list. Waiting for a new lung is a terrible thing because while the patient needs that lung to live, the only way that they can receive a healthy lung is for someone else to pass away. The worst day of someone else's life becomes their best day as one person dies so that they can live. It is both tragic and miraculous all at the same time. However, in this case, the patient's mother knew that she didn't just want to wait around for the death of her own son or that of someone else, so she started researching and found a study in another country on stem cells that her son qualified for. He entered the study and after only receiving the stem cells three times was able to return to work. Truly amazing! Imagine being at death's door and then within three treatments being able to return to life as normal. I was shocked at the results of the majority of the patients in this particular study.

Not only can stem cells adapt, differentiating into other types of cells, but stem cells are also self-propagating which is just a fancy way of saying that they multiply or reproduce. They will give rise to a daughter cell (one just like themselves) and then form the type of cells that are needed for that particular tissue. Therefore if placed in the liver...liver cells, kidney...kidney cells, and so forth. Stem cells live for decades in their own little protective environment called a niche. This provides homeostasis for the safety and well being of the cell and provides it with nutrients so it can continue it's remarkable work.

For some of you, this may be a little too many details about types of stem cells. However, many people ask me about stem cell types especially those who are concerned with being injected with stem cells from aborted fetal cells, so I like to be very clear when I explain this as well as what kind of cells I do and do not use in my practice. Potency is the ability of the stem cell to differentiate or become various types of other cells. There are different types of stem cells and therefore different potencies. Stem cells are classified into five potency categories.

1. Totipotent- These cells can differentiate into any embryonic and extraembryonic cell types. These come from embryonic cells

2. Pluripotent- Descendants of totipotent cells. They can form any cell line from the germ layers. Human embryonic cells form from the blastocyst (conception days 5-14).

3. Multipotent- These are of most interest to us as they form multiple cell types. Easy to get, because they can come from adult stem cells such as fat or bone marrow. They can also come from placenta cord blood and the less desirable amniotic fluid.

4. Oligopotent- These can only differentiate into a few cell types. They can come from the myeloid cells and lymphoid cell lines.

5. Unipotent- These can only produce one cell

line or type, that is like itself. This would be muscle stem cells.

Pluripotent stem cells have the most capabilities for differentiation which sounds wonderful in theory, but there are great ethical considerations. Personally, being a devout believer in Yeshua, I can not bring myself to use these types of cell lines on any individual. Aside from the moral implications of using these cell lines, there is also data from abroad that tells us of frequent dangerous ethical implications from their use including that these pluripotent cells can cause an immune response as well as consistent correlation with the use of the cells and the development of teratomas (tumors). I tend to think of it as God's protection over these embryonic cells that they do have these side effects that make them less than ideal as compared to adult, multipotent stem cells.

With the exception of research study, in the United States, the stem cells used are multipotent stem cells. I like working with the multipotent stem cells because they differentiate into many cell lines, but they also have few side effects. This gives us the great benefits for repairing whatever organ system you need help with, without the worry of creating a new problem such as a teratoma or an immune response. These are also commercially available in the United States, but it remains to be seen how they will become regulated by the FDA. This is currently still controversial, therefore a lot of us on the cutting edge of our field are using bone marrow or fat to obtain the same adult mesenchymal stem cells vs. obtaining them commercially. In my clinic, when this is done we will use a flow cytometer to count the cells and view the viability of the cells. This means we have a machine that counts the stem cells and see if they are healthy and living. If they are living and the numbers are good, you have a greater probability of having a triumphant success story.

This just proves the amazing power of stem cells and all the untapped potential that regenerative medicine has yet to discover. This is why it is so important for me to be on the cutting edge in this field, so that I can help my patients find answers to the physical problems that no one has been able to help them with. I relate deeply on a personal level to the frustration of searching for a healing solution and not being able to find it, yet I also believe that sometimes we search to find answers for healing outside the body when all along God had already created the perfect avenue for healing inside our body. Science just is still discovering and learning to utilize what God had already created at the beginning of time through the brilliance and healing powers of stem cells.

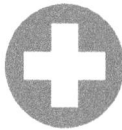

# CHAPTER 11

# Regenerative Medicine: Exosomes

> *Exosomes are noted to carry growth factors that are needed for health and healing as well as proteins that are instrumental in many factors of our health.*

As the field of Regenerative Medicine grows and the study of stem cells evolves and grows along with other cellular therapies; universities, medical centers, and hospitals are rapidly changing to hire specialists in this field. However, this was not always the case. There was a time when I was speaking to a patient about exosomes (cell-derived vesicles) specific for his medical case. When he mentioned these exosomes to his other doctor at a world-renowned medical center, his physician labeled me a quack, told him to stop seeing me as a patient, and denied the existence of exosomes. Therefore, it was quite surprising when the following week he received a call from the same prominent medical center, apologizing and informing him that they had just in fact hired an expert on the subject of exosomes. I was ahead of the curve in my field, but that often left me open to the judgement and harsh criticism of my peers as they clung to more traditional beliefs instead of being open to the constant quest for new knowledge and information.

In my experience as a patient, I had been let down by traditional medicine and the need for practitioners to cling to old ideas instead of branch out, study, and innovate using newer scientific developments in their own practices. This disheartened me as I observed with frustration a failure of traditional doctors endeavoring to learn about and improve their practices and the lives of their patients by grasping on to new innovations and understandings in the field of medicine, but particularly genetics on the cellular level. I frequently saw genetics being misinterpreted and a lacking in physicians dedicated to the understanding of cellular biology and molecular science. Many simply did not have the desire to learn or understand this, but as cells are the building blocks of the body, a clear understanding of them becomes an essential need. I have spent over two hundred and seventy hours studying stem cells, exosomes, platelet-rich plasma (PRP), and other cellular therapies in order to better serve my patients and provide innovative methods of healing and was baffled that even in the medical community there seemed to be a poor understanding of these medical procedures, treatments, and options. As cellular science is a growing and dynamic field, there may be continual changing in our understanding of these things, but it is not beneficial to anyone if we cling to past understandings neglecting to embrace the new knowledge that emerges.

It can be difficult to change the medical community as so many seem to cling to past ideas or hypothesis without considering the scientific changes that have been discovered and are being implemented. One example of this is when we accept scientific hypotheses as facts and do not adjust our thinking as these hypotheses are proven to be incorrect. A prominent illustration of this exists with prostate cancer. In the 1950s a hypothesis was made that testosterone alone leads to prostate cancer and this hypothesis soon became accepted as gospel in relation to this disease. Through developments in science, we now know the causes of prostate cancer can be multifactorial: inherited or acquired genetic mutations, higher levels of androgens, and viruses such as HPV could all be potential contributors. However, based on one hypothesis, testosterone became a controlled substance as the idea that it lead to prostate cancer became medical fact. If anything should be considered as medical fact, it is that our understanding of medical science is an evolving and growing process and we should continue to seek out answers without becoming complacent to accept hypotheses as facts. The Lord made the human body so intricate and complex that lifetimes of study can never fully grasp the understanding of God's marvelous creation.

What precisely are the aforementioned exosomes? Exosomes are nano vesicle particles. That is just a very fancy way of saying that these are very tiny particles that are present in our bodies and are passed between the cells. A Swedish scientist, by the name of Jan Lötvall, discovered that some of these exosomes have a very important job and that is to transfer genetic material from cell to cell-- more specifically messenger ribonucleic acid (RNA) to make proteins and microRNAs to regulate the expression of genes between each other[6]. This meant is that these exosomes had the ability to transfer genetic material from cell to cell in a way that scientists had not fully identified until as recently as 2007.

These messenger RNA are extremely important, because as their name indicates, they communicate between the cells telling them if they need help, are about to expire, or have some beneficial nutrients or particles that can be used for other cells. This transfer of genetic material, however, is a double-edged sword of sorts. Once it was discovered that exosomes could carry genetic material, scientists quickly realized that not only were diseases being spread between the cells by these particles, but they also had the ability to alter the molecules of the exosomes to fight disease and deliver effective genetic therapies. Therefore, exosomes could pass along harmful genetic material or in fact be altered to insert positive genetic therapies. This was an exciting discovery.

Exosomes are noted to carry growth factors that are needed for health and healing as well as proteins that are instrumental in many factors of our health. Anti-inflammatory properties are a key component of these power-packed particles. Often as we age or struggle with chronic disease, these cellular particles do not behave correctly. Exosomes are extremely important because they assist with cell to cell

---

6    (National Cell Biology 2007, Lotvall, DOI: 10.1038/ncb1596)

communication. Correcting the biological pathways that are working incorrectly, through the use of genetic alteration of the exosomes as our cells renew to bring life, and stimulating correct transcription is what I believe what shows the most promise. This possibly offers even greater promise than the use of stem cells especially for an individual with an incorrect genetic expression. Hopefully, through all of our advances, we can streamline the process and make is dually effective by combining the use of stem cell exosomes and gene splicing to provide the best outcome for all individuals.

One of the largest drawbacks to the entire field of regenerative medicine is the lack of finances available to do appropriate double-blind studies to see what are the best modalities for the use of these cellular products. Large studies of this kind are extremely expensive and getting the FDA approval for a product can cost anywhere between eighteen million to over $490,000,000. If the projected end result is that we do not have a product that is a pharmaceutical that can be resold on the market for a lot of money, then the industry won't invest in a study for it. The pharmaceutical industry is the only conglomerate that has pockets deep enough to fund these kinds of studies. Right now there are a small amount of patient funded studies, but the numbers are minimal. We need a larger sampling of numbers to see the true benefit of these cellular products. Hopefully we will see pharmaceutical companies that are willing to advance the field and invest in these studies as exosomes are already showing promise as attractive drug delivery systems.

Daily, I like to review current studies, both here in the United States and abroad. Some of the studies done so far do not show statistical significance, but I believe it is because of the population chosen or the sampled numbers were too small. As I read sources such as *Mesenchymal Cell News*, *Cell Therapy News*, and *Human Immunology News*, I begin to understand the true benefits of cellular therapies. Stem cells, exosomes, PRP, are all showing promise and have helped a significant number of individuals. Although not everyone is helped by these therapies, I believe we can determine why. As diet plays such an integral role in correct gene expression, it is my theory that perhaps the diet was not maximized for effectiveness or they didn't have the adequate nutrients in their system to aid these sophisticated cellular therapies.

Observing miracles that have changed lives inspires me to continue to search and gain more knowledge in this field. I get excited about the possibilities when I witnessed case studies in which for example, an individual who was wheelchair bound and devastated by a genetic disease underwent cellular therapies in conjunction with some concurrent treatments and begin to walk. What an amazing thing for someone who was wheelchair bound to be up and ambulating. To be able to view this occurrence in person was transformative. I have seen the hand of God do miraculous things and I believe this was also one. For some time now, my prayer has been that God will give me wisdom with each patient so I can deliver the best possible medicine for that individual. I want to allow God to do His will through me so that others can see His miraculous hand and be forever changed. He has blessed me with the scholarly desire to always learn more to discover what I can integrate into my practice and through this, I can help to bless and change the lives of as many patients as possible.

Exosomes are just one exciting new branch of study that I can see being of benefit to my patients. If they can carry molecules that can spread disease, then scientists can alter them for use in preventing disease. For example, if exosomes are responsible for distributing the materials that cause plaques to occur in the brains of those with Alzheimer's then it is logical that we can utilize this same distribution method to alter them and in fact provide healing agents to those afflicted with Alzheimer's. The implications for this are so exciting and hopefully, we will see further testing carried out as well as advancements in this field. Stay tuned as I believe that the future role of these tiny genetic transfer players is going to be big!

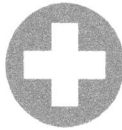

# CHAPTER 12

# Peptide Therapies: The many benefits of infused amino acids.

> *As a physician who has directly benefited and seen my patients benefit from peptides, my goal is to utilize as many of them as possible and stay on the cutting edge in my field to continue to help my patients.*

My own journey with pain led me to find healing, in part, due to what is known as a tripeptide, composed of three amino acids (cysteine, glutamic acid, and glycine) called glutathione. Glutathione is an essential ingredient that just about everyone needs for improved health, but for me, it made the difference between unbearable leg pain and living life again. I believe that everyone would benefit from the use of glutathione and have therefore poured over two thousand hours researching this titan of tripeptides. Genetically speaking, approximately eighteen percent of the population has a difficult time creating cysteine and therefore will be challenged in efforts to produce glutathione.

Glutathione is I what I believe to be our Master antioxidant, as it controls over four hundred functions in our bodies and effects or enables many bodily functions. It is also critical in allowing for other peptides to function correctly. Acting as an immune modulator, glutathione is essential in helping other peptides reach their maximum potential. Understanding the intricacies of peptides and biological functions as well as the interrelationships between peptides is crucial for our overall health.

Peptides are amino acid chains that are shorter than proteins as they are smaller than chains of fifty amino acids, but greater than chains of two amino acids. We have over seven thousand various peptides in our bodies. The peptides help to direct biological pathways in our bodies. They also help our bodies to interpret how our own DNA is read and are therefore critical to our health and wellbeing. Following the age of twenty-one, the peptides that naturally occur in our body start to decline and injecting them it is one way that we can help to heal the breakdown of our cells.

The term peptide might sound strange or unfamiliar to many of you, but you are probably very familiar with insulin which is actually a peptide hormone used most commonly to treat diabetes. Insulin was first used on a human in 1922, to treat diabetes and is still in use today. Like insulin, other peptides have met with much acclaim when approval is granted as they have little to no negative side effects. Usually too small to be absorbed via digestion through pill form, they are most often injected directly into the cells themself.

Predicted to be an over forty-five billion dollar therapeutic drug industry within the next five years, peptides seem to be the new buzz word, but how effective really are they? Sold in everything from eyeliner, to lotion, lipstick, to all manner of make-up and marketed with catchy phrases like "botox in a bottle," "breast booster," "sagging skin serum;" it seems as if it is a cosmetic, it now includes a peptide along with a giant markup in price. Do these products actually work? Given the administering method, it is unlikely, but that is not the case with those in the medical field and this time "Big Pharma" knows that the leaders in integrative medicine are ahead of the game in utilizing these chains of amino acids and they want to cash in. Therefore, they are already investing in the research and development of peptides for medical application in a big way which in turn could be very beneficial for the consumer.

As a physician who has directly benefited and seen my patients benefit from peptides, my goal is to utilize as many of them as possible and stay on the cutting edge in my field to continue to help my patients. The wife of a seventy-two year old male patient of mine brought her husband in to see me. He had been suffering from prostate cancer and had undergone a prostatectomy. The first time I met *Simon*, his pallor was what stood out. It was almost grey as if he was close to death. His wife had desperately wanted him to see me--almost even more than he did. They were devastated by his illness and I was for them as well. He had been on Lupron for quite some time which was a drug that blocked the production of testosterone in the body in order to attempt to stop or fight the cancer, but it wasn't working. Prior to the prostatectomy Simon had undergone different chemo agents without success, and he and his wife came to me begging for some help. I started him on a peptide called IRGD that was specifically for cancer. When I started him on this, his Prostate Specific Antigen (PSA) level was at a twelve. Typically, a 4.0 or lower is consider normal, so this was three times the highest level of what could be considered normal. At the next check, we brought it down to a level of six and finally his PSA was brought down to a level of three which was considered normal. By this time he was looking and feeling better and was able to be more active. It is amazing what the Lord can do within our own bodies.

In the United States at this time, we currently have about thirty-six different FDA approved peptides to work with. If you are in Europe, they have over one hundred peptides available for use. Why are there so few approved by the United States right now as compared to other countries? Similar to other drugs and procedures, we do have more stringent processes here than overseas, but also there are not many pharmaceutical companies approved to even compound peptides which therefore makes them incredibly costly and limits the ability to access. Therefore, some athletes have gone to the extreme lengths of getting them from places like China and have unfortunately lost their lives using illegal peptides. The United States may not have as many approved, but at least you know that you are always getting superior purity, as the purity is mandated to be at least ninety-eight percent. It is always better to ensure that you are doing things in the safest way possible. These peptides function in multiple ways depending on the type of peptide it is. Some have a variety of functions and treat a variety of conditions, while some seem to serve more specific and focus purposes.

For example, one peptide that we are finding great success with is called Thymosin Alpha-1 (TA1). It is often used to activate various cells of the immune system, stimulating them where they are weakened or impaired to help fight off various infections which physicians are finding incredibly useful in the case of cancer patients whose immune systems need help fighting off attacks from other sources of sickness. TA1 also helps to modulate the immune system for those with autoimmune diseases. We know that autoimmune disorders are disorders caused by overactive immune systems attacking our own bodies to devastating effect. These are just a few successful functions of this multi-talented peptide. TA1 is a peptide that is showing great promise for many individuals who have failed other treatment modalities and I have personally born witness to the life-changing effects of this peptide for a variety of my patients. Often used by oncologists in conjunction with chemotherapy, to offset the deprivation in the immune system caused by these treatments. This is a great relief to physicians in the field as chemo often causes deaths due to the weakening and compromisation immune system which is prone to collateral damage that can lead to pneumonia or other killer secondary infections. In my own experience, I have seen several women undergoing breast cancer treatments offset secondary infections due to this powerful peptide.

There is another wonderful peptide known as Thymosin Beta-4 (TB4) which is used for repair of muscles, tendons, ligaments, inflammation and wound healing. Each peptide is unique and therefore each protocol for treatment varies as well. Whereas a peptide treatment for repair with (TB4) might require only one to three injections, a round of (TA1) for someone with breast cancer might require daily at-home injections for six months.

As a former OB/GYN, I have seen many parents struggle sexual dysfunction or with infertility and witnessed women struggle through round after round of hormone injections in the desire to conceive. Costs associated with infertility can quickly become budget-breaking as expenses for treatment can rapidly destroy finances while simultaneously taking its toll on the human body. Fertility costs for methods such as in vitro are often prohibitive to those couples on a more limited budget. A peptide known as Kisspeptin-10 is changing that. Known as a regulator of the reproductive system, it helps stimulate and increase the luteinizing hormone in both men and women signaling reproduction and is showing great potential abroad. The costs associated with the use of this peptide are significantly lower than those with more invasive procedures. There are additional peptides that work optimizing low spermatogenesis in men and while others promote the follicle-stimulating hormone to maximize its effectiveness. It is very exciting to be able to offer peptides that can bring forth life with less difficulty and personal cost to those facing fertility challenges.

The variety in the functions of peptides is amazing. Although we might not have as many approved here in the United States as there are in Europe for example, there still is such a huge variety in peptides that there seems to be one available for most conditions. I also find them very beneficial to use in my practice as they do not have issues with interacting in a negative way with other treatments. Most of my patients do not have one simple issue, they have a complex case of issue and therefore require several forms of treatments and peptides do not interfere with this. I am able to give someone IV treatments while simultaneously treating them with the appropriate peptide.

For example, another physician brought her daughter, *Abigail*, to see me. She was seventeen years old and had been diagnosed with Crohn's disease. Her healthy weight had been around 127 pounds, but now after being sick, she weighed a mere eighty-four pounds. She had been in and out of the hospital, unable to tolerate any food and actually had a nutritional IV line. Her treatment took place on multiple fronts. First I started to give her a peptide injection to promote gut healing. This particular peptide is known as BPC-157 and has been proven to repair the gut. I have seen amazing success with it within my own practice and even with my own daughter's aforementioned weeping rash associated with zonulin. This particular peptide is available in both injection and pill form, but as Abigail was not tolerating much of anything in her stomach, I chose the injection. After that began to work, I switched her to the pill form and within five weeks she was able to tolerate food again. She had gone from fifteen bowel movements a day all the way down to three and begin to gain healthy weight back again.

During her testing, I evaluated Abigail as having mold toxicity and it was discovered that she and her mom had been living in a moldy house. Therefore, while she was being treated with peptides she was also to undergo IV treatments along with her mother to address the mold toxicity issue.

Not only did BPC-157 help heal Abigail, stabilized for oral consumption it is now being used in many patients with gastrointestinal distress, Crohn's, Colitis, or IBS and has exhibited much success. In injectable form, it is also used for muscle, tendon, and ligament repair and has shown many benefit in these areas.

Another one of my patients had a truly amazing healing story with this particular peptide. Her

name was *Olivia*. She was thirty-four and a mother
of three children who developed Crohn's disease
after mold exposure. Previously prescribed multiple
medications including Humira, she had begun
having side effects due to the medication including
increased fatigue, hair loss, and the inability to
focus. Needing to work while having cognitive
functions at maximum capacity, Olivia began
to seek alternative treatments for managing her
Crohn's disease. After a full laboratory work-up
and medical assessment, to make sure that she
didn't have any additional or underlying problems,
we proceeded to work towards getting her Crohn's
under control. Malnourished and cachectic, Crohn's
had caused significant weight loss that leached her
body of nutritional resources. We worked together
to replace the nutritional deficit and began using
peptide therapy first treating her with a series of
TA1 followed by BPC-157, first in subcutaneous
injections and finally on the stabilized form for
oral consumption in order to bring healing to
her gastrointestinal tract. Once her body began
producing healthy stool outputs, Olivia began to
state that she was having less pain and her energy
was increasing as well. Soon she was able to
discontinue her biologics and upon stopping her
other medication her hair began to regrow and she
states at this time that she now "has a new lease on
life."

Olivia is just one of many patients that have
been helped with peptide therapy and autoimmune

or gastrointestinal distress. It is amazing to see patients participate in life again. These individuals can now participate in family events, work a normal functioning job, and once again feel like a contributing member of society. Given my own experience, I know how incredible that is.

Another fantastic peptide of great interest to me which has been used widely in Europe and even more extensively in Russia is called Epithalon. Used after Chernobyl to assist in undoing some of the effects of radiation poisoning, in America Epithalon is known as a telomere lengthener. A telomere is a section of DNA extending from the end of our chromosomes and they are responsible for protecting our genetic information, helping cells divide and their length of an individual's telomeres dictates an individual's lifespan. Therefore, Epithalon is known as a lifespan extender. The longer our telomeres are, it seems our capacity to resist disease is greater...especially those diseases related to aging. Since aging is a known disease state, this peptide can reduce aging. This peptide also has neuroendocrine regulatory responses which means that it can help regulate a person's neuronal response to the endocrine glands which control metabolism growth and development. Since the endocrine system also helps regulate our sleep, mood, and other similar functions, there has been some positive results reported with Epithalon assisting in restoring the circadian rhythm and allowing for increased sleep function.

When a patient comes to me for treatment, it is not a guessing game as to which peptide I will treat them with. I give them a complete physical, review their lab values, their genetic evaluations, and the patient's symptoms to choose the peptide plan that is correct for them.

Certain peptides are showing tremendous results for cognitive dysfunction such as early Alzheimer's and other neurological diseases such as Parkinson's. These peptides particularly help in slowing down the decline of secondary symptoms associated with their disease state. For an individual to be able to live a longer period of time without the devastating side effects of cognitive decline and immobility, these changes brought by peptides are indispensable in the eyes of the patient's family and loved ones.

Recently I had another patient named, *Jimmy*, a seventy-eight-year-old male struggling with Parkinson's disease. Diagnosed at the age of fifty-seven, he spent many years doing well with traditional medications as he enjoyed life as a happily married man, blessed with four children and sixteen grandchildren. Eventually, after years of medication, he had suddenly seemed to become resistant to the medication and was not getting the same results. He had noticed that a few hours after it was time to take his medication, his symptoms would grow dramatically worse. His feet would shuffle and drag, his face would lose expressions and he would get tremors in his hands. In fact, within two hours of taking the medicine, he would already be struggling with rigidity and walking. Since he was only seventy-eight, he was not ready to slow down in life, but also did not want to invest in any large scale treatment options. His wife had additionally noted that he was struggling cognitively. She reported that he had always been a great conversationalist and would enjoy talking over a cup of tea, but now was struggling to retain the skills to carry on a conversation. She was distraught, because he seemed to be slipping away from her. After fully evaluating him and discussing his situation with him, together we decided that his best option would be to try to alternate two different peptides, Semax and Selank, that were to be given intranasally. Our plan was to alternate these peptides so that he would have the ability to go for longer periods of unaffected time between his Parkinson's medicine dosages. Six weeks later, he came back ecstatic. He could walk normally, his face appeared completely normal and he exhibited no tremors in his hands. Amazingly, not only was he able to go longer between medication dosages without the accompanying fatigue, tremors, or foot shuffling, but his wife reported joyfully that his cognitive function returned and he was able to carry on conversations and go on outdoor walks again. I noticed a huge change as well and where I had initially seen him exhibiting the "mask" or facial appearance that eventually affects most Parkinson's patients, the mask had lifted and I was overjoyed to see this dear man with expression and enthusiasm for life. It is my desire to help everyone to be able to enjoy their life to the fullest.

My patients get so excited when they are healed, but I also rejoice with them. I know what it is like to rely on others to search and not find answers and that is why I have dedicated my life to finding answers for my patients. This is why when I first started hearing about peptides outside of the traditional medical uses such as insulin for diabetes or oxytocin for childbirth, I took the time to investigate it and learn more.

Oddly enough, I first heard about peptides being used for healing in the fitness center or gym setting as they had been traditionally used for athletes working to develop strength and endurance. A lot of non-FDA approved supplement type products get their starts here. Therefore, I thought that I would research the science behind some of these peptides that were being talked about. This led to my attendance at a conference for both integrative and traditional doctors taught by Dr. Seeds of the Cleveland Clinic. At the time, there were maybe ten total peptides used in the United States, but this conference vaulted me into a different level of knowledge about peptides. This began my a whole new level of understanding for me in the world of peptides and I continued to devote time and research into learning more ways to use them and apply them in my practice. Now I get asked to speak at conferences throughout the country about peptides, because of my continued advancement in this field.

When speaking, I often get asked what the FDA's stance on peptide therapy. Unfortunately, they have not made clear a stance on the majority of peptides at this point. A few have been relegated to a "do not compound list," but there are approximately seven thousand peptides currently under development and very few have been crossed over to clinical application at this point. Many peptides, including those in other countries, are still being used mainly as research bases. At this point, most peptides are being governed by individual states and the pharmacy boards of those states which greatly limits their use and access in certain states. Due to this, it is difficult for many in the United States to utilize peptides that could make a significant change in the status of their health. As peptides continue to gain status in the more innovative fringes of medicine, rulings will be made before too long on the use of each individual peptide. In May of 2017, President Donald Trump signed the "Right to Try" Act which has permitted many patients the ability to try medications not yet FDA approved as well as alternative therapies not approved by traditional Western medicine. Even with this Act in place, there are still rules and guidelines that must be followed according to state governing boards.

It is my opinion that understanding peptides is critical in understanding cellular health. Without a complete understanding of cellular health, it is impossible to fully treat overall developing health. Recent research has found that there are over 270 peptides which affect the mitochondria in our body. The mitochondria are a critical part of each of the trillions of cells in our body and biotoxin disease, autoimmune disorders, aging, and a multitude of diseases that can damage these integral cellular structures. Through the use of peptides, we can undo these effects damaging the mitochondria and work toward actually healing the mitochondria. I don't believe that the future for the attainment of peptides to specifically heal mitochondria is that far away and the implications of that should be exciting for all.

Peptides are the future of medicine and increased cellular health and therefore it is exciting to be at the forefront of this medical expedition and to be able to witness the amazing results from their use, brought forth in the lives of my patients. I can't wait to see what else is in store for this game-changing use of these power-packed amino acid chains, but I am confident that the use of peptides will continue to be life-changing for my patients.

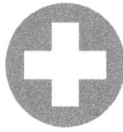

# CHAPTER 13

# The Spiritual Effects of Illness

*I believe that there is no part of our physical creation that is not interdependent and this includes our spirit and soul. This interdependence means that our body can affect our spirit and our soul and vice versa.*

When we cause our own spirit to be subjected to the spirit of God, our spirit is in communication with God. Our spirit is the part of us that is redeemed when salvation occurs. Our soul, mind, will, and emotions the personality will become a conduit of the spirit man. Romans 12:2 states, *"do not be conformed to the pattern of this world, but be transformed by the renewing of our mind."* We must take every thought captive in order to renew our minds. It is imperative that we do not allow our minds to dictate inappropriate actions or wrongness in our thought life. We must meditate on the things of the Lord, as it is the Word of God that brings the renewing of the mind.

The body is the reflection of our outward actions and often our bodies are where the attacks from the world manifest in true illness as we fall prey to a fallen world. The law of the Old Testament was put into place to dictate and control our outward actions. We understand that through the law, we as sinners can not keep the commands of a righteous God. Through Jesus Christ, our spirit is renewed and born again.

You may be wondering where I am going with this or questioning how this topic has anything to do with a particular illness or pertain to your personal goal of wellness and healing? I assure you that it is extremely relevant. Many times within my practice, I have encountered patients who do not get well even though from a medical standpoint it seems that they are healed. Often their numbers have improved while we have removed the many toxins that have caused inflammation or other contributors to illness. In my years of examining these phenomena--patients who by all standards seem to be healed, but still complain of illness when nothing measurable exists, I often find the same patient correlations. When investigated in-depth, I realize that these patients had their own set of common denominators: including a very low self-esteem, an attitude of ever-present despair, and the inability to control their tongue in the sense that they speak negativity over their lives. I believe that these factors equate to essentially illness spoken over and into the lives of these patients every hour of the day to the detriment of their own healing.

I would like to tell you this story to better illustrate what I am attempting to portray. *Janel* is a forty-six year-old female who became ill from various infective agents including the Epstein-Barr virus. Additionally, she had been diagnosed through traditional medicine with fibromyalgia and chronic fatigue. After unsuccessfully trying many medications typically available for those illnesses and failing, she came to see me. We discussed many factors including Epstein-Barr as well as some of the other bacterial and viral agents possibly leading to her current state of illness. As part of our treatment plan, I instructed her that I wanted her to speak positive affirmations into the mirror while she simultaneously looked herself in the eyes. I found this practice to be relevant because if we are voicing either healing scriptures or positive affirmations and we cannot look at our self in the eye then we typically do not believe that those words are for us. She agreed to do this along with the planned treatments. Once the treatment began, she struggled to get through it. However, in the end, I was ecstatic as she now tested with negative results for the Epstein-Barr virus as well as some of the other viral elements and bacterial elements found in our exam and labs including Bartonella. Post-treatment, Janel continued to complain of the same exact symptoms as she had before, but all of her labs were completely normal. This included all of her inflammatory markers and any markers for chronic inflammatory response (CIRS). Her spouse even reported to me that she seemed to be moving around better and able to do more than before, however, he also observed that she continually spoke sickness and illness over herself and her body. This was quite concerning to him because he saw the possibility of her getting well, but meanwhile, she was refusing to speak health into her body and it seemed was, therefore, holding herself hostage in a state of illness. This is one of many examples that I have seen where individuals seem to be healed, but continue to speak sickness over themselves and their bodies and therefore never get truly well. Our soul, mind, will, and emotions can speak negativity that will affect our body and our spirit as well. Our spirit cannot grow when we are speaking evil and death into our own lives.

In general, integrative medicine takes a very holistic and whole-body approach to understand the effects of illness on the body. I believe that there is no part of our physical creation that is not interdependent and this includes our spirit and soul. This interdependence means that our body can affect our spirit and our soul and vice versa. This is why I love for us, as individuals, to practice speaking through the Spirit in submission to God, submitting our body and soul to the Holy Spirit. If we command our triune being or nature to be under the authority of God then we have the ability to walk in wholeness.

This does not discredit the sovereignty of God as He is all-powerful and omniscient, or all knowing. We will never know or understand why some individuals are completely healed instantaneously, others have a process to their healing, and some only receive healing through death. We live in a fallen world and cannot control that and we also cannot control God. Many of us are trying to control God by being good, being diligent, and following rituals or behavior that we think is correct, but God is sovereign and we cannot dictate to him. We can not earn His favor. It is freely given. My wife once posted this message on social media, "We do what's right because we have a relationship with God, not to get a relationship with Him." We do what is right because of our love for Him, not to try and get healing or earn something from Him. If nothing else, we have already received the most important thing, salvation. We have eternal life because of what Jesus did for us.

I often observe Christians behaving in a way that is judgmental, unforgiving, and controlling, yet it is unbelievable that we as mere humans would try to control the all-powerful God. We cannot control God. We love God so much because of what he has done for us. Even if our healing is not recognized in this world, we have still received such a great miracle in salvation and eternity in Heaven. I see some Christians that are so judgmental that there is a complete lack of love. This lack of love is not conducive to healing. When the scripture says, "that by His stripes we are healed," this is not out of a spirit of judgment, but out of love. The Word of God says that if we do not forgive we cannot be forgiven. I have seen time and time again that those with unforgiveness become extremely bitter. This bitterness will lead to unbelievable health problems. Is this why the church is so sick today? In my personal life, I have had many Christians wrong me. In fact, some have done things to wrong me only to turn around and blame me for doing something to them. What is the right thing to do in that situation? I have chosen to forgive them when they wronged me and have humbled myself to them even though they had accused me of causing offense that was untrue. When we take a spirit of love, forgiveness, and humility, this opens up the door for the healing of our body, mind, and spirit.

It is my desire that we all walk in health and healing. Unfortunately, this will not always happen, but nevertheless, we should still keep on attempting to find health and healing for all. Personally, I want to help individuals find healing through their bodies, which includes healing the words spoken from their mouth. The mouth speaks forth words that are positive or negative which gives a vibration of good or bad to those nearby. We are created in the image of God. God spoke the world into existence just as we can speak life or death. The Word of God tells us in Proverbs 18:21, "Death and life are in the power of the tongue." We can choose to speak life to ourselves and to others. We can control our tongue by controlling our mind as well and we must bring every thought captive. The captivity of our mind is controlled by the Word of God which brings forth life. I pray that we may all have life and life abundantly. This is my prayer for you today.

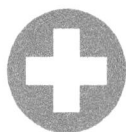

# Epilogue

I've always recommended my patients to take daily supplements. I do this, in part, because I know how much daily supplements helped me recover and stay healthy. In fact, when I forget to take my daily supplements, I immediately start feeling more lethargic!

Taking daily supplements is an easy way to stay on top of your health goals, and avoid a costly illness in the future. But knowing which supplements to take is the hard part...until now. I began to research genetic testing as it relates to daily supplements, then working with my patients I learned how genetic testing could be the answer to helping discover the best supplements to take for your unique health issues.

Scientists recently acknowledged that variations in our genes determine how well our bodies metabolize certain compounds and vitamins. This means that for some people, they are literally taking the wrong supplements for their individual DNA make-up. What a terrible waste of money!

How does knowing your genetic makeup help you in the long run? Your lab results and body metrics will give you a better insight on what your body needs more of, can do without, and what you can do to help prevent potential diseases and other health risks.

For example, I can create a personalized nutrition plan based on your DNA results. I can show you which medications to avoid and which medications to take. Best of all, I can show you which daily supplements will help you and which ones might actually harm you. Once you know this information, you can fine tune your nutrition, exercise and supplement routine for improved support. Some of my patients tell me that my supplement recommendations have literally changed their lives. They feel healthier and have more energy.

Knowing your genetic makeup may be a relatively new way to better assess the kinds of vitamins and supplements your body needs, but as it continues to evolve there will be more support for those wanting to live a healthy lifestyle. Whether you choose to modify your diet for optimal energy and support and make more informed supplement decisions, certain DNA tests may help you live your life to the fullest.

I've also developed and created daily supplements that are 100% pure and all-natural. As you read earlier in this book, I discourage people from buying their supplements at grocery stores or drug stores. These supplements often contain synthetic substances and are almost always imbalanced. So through my own research, collaborating with other Integrative physicians, and in working with my patients, I offer a variety of daily supplements. You may take these supplements with or without my DNA test, but you will see the best results after we look at your lab work and genetics.

## Intracellular MTHFR

Some individuals have a genetic mutation which prohibits the proper absorption of Vitamin B. This leads to a general lack of energy, premature aging, and eventually chronic disease. Some people complain of cognitive issues including inability to focus and even depression or anxiety. Intracellular MTHFR is designed specifically for this individual who is heterozygous or homozygous for the C677T or A1298C and is under-methylating (has little or no COMT or MAO) and needs more methylation support. Dr. Crozier recommends this supplement for his patients whose DNA has been tested and who have this specific glitch in their DNA, and also for patients who take a Vitamin B but with no positive health benefits.

## Mitochondrial B12

Dr. Crozier discovered this powerful B12 supplement which transforms B12 into energy at the mitochondrial level. He recommends this supplement to patients who have been diagnosed with chronic fatigue and fibromyalgia, and other chronic conditions which include an extreme lack of energy. This is also an ideal supplement for individuals who have a high homocysteine level, also called hyperhomocysteinemia, which can contribute to arterial damage and blood clots in your blood vessels. Mitochondrial B12 contains 3000 mcg of vitamin B12 in its pure adenosylcobalamin form. Adenosylcobalamin is considered an active coenzyme form of B12, meaning it is used directly in B12-dependent enzyme reactions in the body.

## Cellular Botanical Support

This unique blend of botanical extracts used for centuries to support a healthy gastrointestinal microbial balance, now available as a daily supplement. There are 16 specific herbal substances in this one supplement pill, which all combined provide you with a powerful, natural cleansing agent and particularly for individuals who have gastrointestinal issues or a "leaky gut." Dr. Crozier's patients with Lyme Disease and mold toxicity benefit from this herbal supplement because the disease often results in an imbalance in the gut, preventing nutrients from reaching and healing the body. If you are facing any issues relating to your gastrointestinal system or nutrition, this is an ideal supplement to add to your daily regimine.

## Cellular Neuronal Health

Developed for Dr. Crozier's patients who are experiencing neurological and related mental disorders including depression and anxiety, this powerful combination of key vitamins, minerals, plant extracts, and amino acids support proper neurological function. The amino acids in this unique supplement are blended with specific plant extracts that helps augment neurological health at the level of the neurotransmitter receptor (also known as a neuroreceptor), targeting the cells and providing the patient with relief without dangerous side-effects often associated with pharmaceuticals. This supplement is also a great anti-aging supplement for brain health.

## Cellular Tri Digest

Proper digestive function is a critical element to health and healing, and also to anti-aging. The problem for many people is after a lifetime of ingesting and digesting processed foods, the digestive tract becomes unbalanced and is unable to properly support the body's need for nutrients. This supplement is a powerful, comprehensive blend of enzymes, herbs, and other targeted nutrients to help restore and support digestive function. Dr. Crozier recommends this supplement for all his patients who are over age 40, those who are working on better weight management, and those who need to better synthesize their fats, carbs, and proteins to get maximum potential from the food they eat.

## Cellular Detox Catalase

Finally, one supplement combining two important antioxidants, Superoxide Dismutase and Catalase. When excessive amount of destructive free radicals, including Super Oxide and hydrogen peroxide, are not quenched in your body, they can profilterate into dangerous compounds including peroxynitrite, resulting in physiological changes may induce CFS symptoms including fatigue, immune dysfunction, learning and memory dysfunction, multi-organ pain, exercise intoler-ance, even certain cancers. Dr. Crozier's patients benefit from this supplement as the enzymes are important for neutralization of destructive free radicals. It will help you to detox and restore at the cellular level.

## Intracellular Detox Assist

Glutathione is one of the body's most important and potent antioxidants, and while most antioxidants are found in the foods you eat, glutathione is produced by your body. Unfortunately our bodies produce less glutathione as we age. This important supplement is designed to support individuals with the CBS variant, or other physiological causes, that limit the production of cysteine and sulfur to produce our body's most powerful antioxidant, glutathione. It also contains glycine, which can be necessary when individuals have the SHMT variant or are low on glycine from their diet. It will help your body to recirculate and create glutathione at the intra-cellular level. Dr. Crozier often recommends this supplement for his Lyme and mold toxicity patients.

## Double Nitro Production

Designed specifically for those with the NOS enzyme variant or variants that lower BH4, and for those patients who may experience symptoms of low nitric oxide production such as hypertension, cold hands and feet, and/or erectile dysfunction. This supplement contains rich nutrients and an herbal combination that support the NOS enzyme, which supports the conversion of L-arginine into nitric oxide. This is Dr. Crozier's preferred supplement to help you pump more blood and get more oxygen to your muscles! If you are a beginning or experienced weight trainer or if you exercise, you will want to work this supplement into your daily regimen. It's a great way to help you with your cardio and especially for sexual dysfunction.

## Cellular Amino Complete

Many individuals take a daily Vitamin C supplement, which is necessary for the growth, development, and repair of all body tissues. But most Vitamin C supplements are made from synthetic substances which either don't absorb into your body or, even worse, can make you sick. Dr. Crozier's preferred Vitamin C supplement is pure and all-natural. The benefits are important and long-lasting. It will help support your immune system, adrenal function, collagen formation for healthy skin, and cardiovascular health. Remember your body does not make vitamin C, so it must be taken in through diet or supplementation. This is a "must" for anyone fighting disease. Beware of Vitamin C imitations you see online or at stores!

## DAO Cellular Sensitivity

Dr. Crozier's unique histamine scavenger is a unique formulation used to help the body clear itself of excess histamine. Histamine is a compound which is released by cells in response to injury and in allergic and inflammatory reactions, causing contraction of smooth muscle and dilation of capillaries. Histamine can be generated from acute or chronic inflammation and has many unpleasant downstreams effects on the body. Gut dysbiosis can also generate histamine that further impairs digestion. This product is designed to help scavenge excess histamine in the body and pairs well with APB1 Assist for complete histamine metabolism, as well as Histamine Balancer Liquescence for proper desensitization. Individuals with an overreaction to environmental toxins often produce too much Histamine, which makes this an especially helpful supplement.